# A Practical Guide to Care Planning in Health and Social Care

# A Practical Guide to Care Planning in Health and Social Care

Marjorie Lloyd

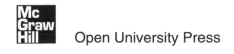

Open University Press

Open University Press
McGraw-Hill Education
McGraw-Hill House
Shoppenhangers Road
Maidenhead
Berkshire
England
SL6 2QL

email: enquiries@openup.co.uk
world wide web: www.openup.co.uk

and Two Penn Plaza, New York, NY 10121—2289, USA

First published 2010

A catalogue record of this book is available from the British Library

ISBN-10: 0-33-523732-0 (pb) 0-33-523731-2 (hb)
ISBN-13: 978-0-33-523732-6 (pb) 978-0-33-523731-9 (hb)

Library of Congress Cataloging-in-Publication Data
CIP data applied for

Typeset by Kerrypress Ltd, Luton, Bedfordshire
Printed and bound in the UK by Bell and Bain Ltd., Glasgow

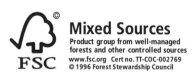

**Mixed Sources**
Product group from well-managed
forests and other controlled sources
www.fsc.org Cert no. TT-COC-002769
© 1996 Forest Stewardship Council

*The McGraw·Hill Companies*

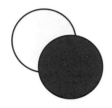

# Praise for this book

"Those of us who work in health or social care need to both understand and reflect upon the care decisions we make. We must be able to account for our practice and justify our decisions in a cogent and transparent way. Marjorie Lloyd logically and persuasively demonstrates the importance of this process in ensuring the best possible outcomes for patients and clients in our care. In support of the author's own plea, this book should be used both wisely and well."

Tonks Fawcett, University of Edinburgh, UK

"A structured plan is the essential foundation for the delivery of safe and effective care. This publication successfully guides the reader through the stages of care planning using a simple yet systematic approach. Its strength lies in the carefully designed format which gives consideration to the evidence base as well as providing guidance for the practical application of care plans. A valuable resource which will capture the interest of all those involved in planning high quality care."

Carol Dickie, University of the West of Scotland, UK

"This is an excellent book for anyone starting out on the Common Foundation year of their nursing degree, and as a reference to those further into their degree, on placement, or newly qualified. The care planning process is very well introduced using models and frameworks of care, with thorough explanations and visual aids ... I would have no hesitation in recommending this book to fellow students and colleagues, and I will use it through the remainder of my degree and beyond."

Conor Hamilton, Student Nurse, Queens University Belfast, UK

# Contents

**You can find printable downloads of all practice sheets online at:**
**www.openup.co.uk/careplanning**

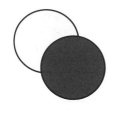

# Introduction: why do we need a book on care planning?

*We need a more personalized NHS, responsive to each of us as individuals, focused upon prevention, better equipped to keep us healthy and capable of giving us real control and real choices over our lives.*

(Prime Minister Gordon Brown, DoH 2008b)

*What the Baby P case calls into question is not so much the structures or systems, more the individual practice. From the paediatrician who allegedly failed to identify the toddler's probably fractured ribs and broken spine to the social workers and health visitors who appear to have accepted excuses for the lesser but regular injuries, the tragic story points to a reticence on the part of professionals to investigate, question and challenge.*

(Brindle 2008)

Some people might argue that caring is the most natural thing in the world, so why do we need a book on how to do it? However, those of us who have chosen caring as a profession must be able to account for our practice to those who pay us to do so and the vulnerable people in our care. The above quotes provide examples of how and why health and social care services *must* change. In today's western society, people expect good quality care and are deeply shocked when it is not delivered. It could be argued that there is no excuse for poor practice. However, human beings will always be at risk of making poor judgements for a variety of reasons, one being the fact that we are emotional beings and are not programmed to work like computers. In health and social care, every day, we have to make decisions about our own actions and the actions of others, which will include managing risk to some extent. It is impossible to eliminate all risks but it is not impossible to be able to identify what they are and to address them in some way or another.

The one tool that we will all be familiar with in practice, if not in our own care, is the *care plan*, which is a way of 'signposting' care and agreeing levels and provision of care. However, very little time is spent in much of the policy and practice literature on this important skill and aspect of practice. The care plan is the linchpin of good quality care because it is there for everyone who needs to see it, documenting what is planned to be done and how it will be carried out. This involves skills in assessment, planning and evaluation, with a keen sense for observing when things are not going according to plan. The creation of the care plan is an important task, and yet many of us complain about the burden of paperwork as if it is meant to be some sort of punishment forced upon us. It is not, and the care plan is our *only* evidence that good quality care is being provided effectively and efficiently. Without the care plan, no one would know what is intended to happen and who is involved in delivering the care.

Some practitioners are used to keeping their own notes and ideas to themselves, but this is becoming increasingly unacceptable in practice and in many fields shared care plans and notes are often required. Care professionals are dependent upon each other to ensure that they have provided all the information needed, in order that important decisions can be made quickly by practitioners in numerous fields. Care plans cover the care needs of each individual in our care, from the elderly to the very young, including those who cannot speak for themselves. It is essential that we strive to deliver the best possible care available and are able to account for every action we take along the way. *A Practical Guide to Care Planning in Health and Social Care* will help you to do just that.

## Who needs a book on care planning?

This book is for undergraduate and foundation degree readers in health and social care courses and will also be of interest to other people involved in care planning, including clients, carers and voluntary sector workers. Care planning has been around for some time in the health and social care professions and in nursing since the 1970s. However, as policy and practice change and develop, care planning has become part of many people's daily activities who are involved in health and social care practices.

Throughout this book, professional codes of conduct and ethical considerations will be identified where applicable in order to point out their relevance. These codes of conduct are usually provided in professional documents for each separate profession and, while available to all, can be difficult to transfer into practice.

We all need to be aware that there are codes of practice to help professionals make important decisions about care provision. Professional skills requirements will also be discussed, including *The National Occupational Standards for Social Work* (Topss 2004), The NHS *Knowledge and Skills Framework* for health care workers (DoH 2004) and the Quality Assurance Agency's *Subject Benchmark Statements for Health and Social Care* (QAA 2006). These are areas of health and social care practice that are relevant to everyone involved in the care planning process. To follow the practical theme of this book they will therefore be identified as their relevance arises in different chapters.

## How to use this book

A multidisciplinary approach will be taken throughout this book in order to reflect current practice initiatives and requirements. In addition, ways of involving the person who is receiving health and social care will be identified using a single case study approach, and values and attitudes that will facilitate involvement and partnership working will be identified. Examples will be provided of an assessment using a fictitious case study of a person called Brian. People such as Brian are often referred to as 'clients' or 'patients' and this book uses these terms interchangeably. The development of the *therapeutic relationship* will also be explored, and the important connection between this and the development of communication skills.

> **Please note:** Brian is a fictitious character suffering from diabetes. He was created to help us explore the care planning process in relation to a person who suffers from an illness that is familiar to most people. However, this book is not about the management of diabetes and does not provide up-to-date information on diabetes care provision. The purpose of introducing Brian is to see how the process of care planning works and you are advised to seek expert opinion on any illness or disease that presents within a particular person's care planning needs.

Each chapter will outline the potential learning outcomes at the beginning and will conclude with a summary of important points to remember and reflect on, followed by an opportunity to test yourself with some self-assessment questions. Sample documentation that may be used in the care planning process is provided throughout the book and copies are to be found in the appendix for students to use to practise the skills involved in documenting a care plan.

To get the full benefit from this book, it should be read in the usual order, from front to back. However, each individual chapter is a useful source in its own right. The chapters are designed to give you all the help you need throughout the care planning process in whatever role you are involved with. You are an important contribution to the quality of health and social care service provision, however great or small your involvement. *For the sake of all the people in your care, please use this book wisely and use it well.*

Chapter 1 introduces the care planning process and provides an overview of that process and the models and frameworks that may be familiar in your own practice. The chapter also introduces an *empowerment model* of care planning for health and social care that puts the client at the centre of the process. This chapter provides a brief overview of the whole care planning process which will be discussed in more detail in the following chapters.

Chapter 2 explores the *assessment* of needs and identifies areas that will be included in the care plan. The skills required to assess need are discussed alongside the policy that guides practice. Practice documentation and reader activities will help you to reflect on your practice and identify barriers to effective assessment. Professional codes of conduct will also be explored in more detail in this and the following chapters.

Chapter 3 introduces *planning* care with the individual in need. The chapter covers how to plan goals, examines barriers to effective planning and explores the role of the multidisciplinary team. You will be encouraged to explore the above in relation to your own areas of practice which may be quite different. Throughout the book you are encouraged to identify key areas of practice relevant to effective and efficient care planning and develop your own practice accordingly. This will include using evidence-based practice and recognizing how to involve clients and carers in the care planning process.

Chapter 4 considers the *implementation* of the care plan so as to facilitate empowerment, emancipation and recovery for the client. *Team working* and the importance of *reflective practice* is emphasized and you will be encouraged to develop you reflective practice skills in order to identify areas of practice that will require further study. The importance of managing the environment and resources will be discussed. Standards of care, cultural diversity and record-keeping will also be emphasized in this chapter. A tool for reflective practice is provided to help you to begin thinking about your practice and the efficiency of the care plan.

Chapter 5 explores the *evaluation* of the care plan, including individual practice. Personal *supervision* will be discussed in more detail as a method of evaluating care individually and in practice. You will be encouraged to use your reflections identified in the previous chapter to explore alternative ways of planning care.

Chapter 6 looks at concluding the care planning process and key recommendations for future practice. This chapter reflects on the process of care planning in health and social care and relates key areas of practice to the clinical and social governance framework that will be discussed further in Chapter 7. The chapter provides an overview of the key characteristics of care planning in health and social care. It also identifies important points for consideration when planning care and provides guidelines for practice in the form of a checklist which can be used in personal supervision sessions with your tutor, manager or mentor.

Chapter 7 explores government and local *policy and law* and introduces you to the roles and responsibilities of the different types of care provision, such as primary care, secondary care, the voluntary and private sectors, social services, clinical and social governance, and their influence on individualized care planning, managers' responsibilities and case note audit. A brief example of how different service providers may influence an individual care plan is given to show how all the different sectors function together.

## Useful resources

At the end of the book you will find a glossary of useful and commonly used terms. There is also a list of recommended reading to help widen your knowledge on the issues touched on in this book but not examined in detail, a selection of useful websites for information and research and finally, following the reference section, an appendix containing samples of the documentation used throughout the book for you to photocopy and use to practise your care planning skills.

# Introduction to the care planning process

## Introduction

*To be faced by a troubled conflicted person who is seeking and expecting help, has always constituted a great challenge to me. Do I have the knowledge, the resources, the psychological strength, the skills – do I have whatever it takes to be of help to such an individual?*

(Rogers 1967: 31)

Every time we are approached for help from individuals or their carers we have to start thinking the same as Carl Rogers thought when he began his psychotherapy practice in the 1960s. However, although there is an expectation on each and every one of us to have some knowledge about what we are doing every day in our practice, more importantly we must know *how* to use that knowledge to obtain the best available help for the people in our care (Schön 1983; Ghaye 2000; Jaspers 2003). Accountability for our practice is increasingly evident in the public reports that result when things go wrong. However, this chapter is not about frightening practitioners into demonstrating good quality care, but is concerned with helping you to be accountable for your practice by making the best use of the processes available to you. The main process in which this can be evidenced is in the *care planning process*, and all practitioners, clients and carers are now expected to have some involvement in care planning. Even if you are not responsible for the whole care plan, knowing how your contribution develops into a good quality plan will help you understand that the process is there to help everyone involved.

## What is care planning?

For those of us involved in health and social care practice and education, care planning affects most of our daily lives. The following professional standards clearly outline the expectations that are placed upon us. In *The Knowledge and Skills Framework* (KSF) (DoH 2004) for health and *The National Occupational Standards for Social Work* (Topss 2004) there is reference to the ability to organize and plan care. For example, the KSF states that at the following levels you should be able to:

- **Level 1:** undertake care activities to meet individuals' health and well-being needs.
- **Level 2:** undertake care activities to meet the health and well-being needs of individuals with a greater degree of dependency.
- **Level 3:** plan, deliver and evaluate care to meet people's health and well-being needs.
- **Level 4:** plan, deliver and evaluate care to meet people's complex health and social care needs.

So at some level, if you work in an environment that provides health care, you must be able to address the health and well-being needs of individual people. For social care workers *The National Occupational Standards* (Topss 2004: 14) state that you should be able to 'Plan, carry out, review and evaluate social care practice with individuals, families, carers' groups, communities and other professionals'. This is also supported by the Quality Assurance Agency (QAA) *Subject Benchmark Statements* in the following areas:

- *the identification and assessment of health and social care needs in the context of individual interaction with their environment;*
- *the development of focused intervention to meet these needs;*
- *implementation of these plans;*
- *critical evaluation of the impact of professional and service interventions on patients and clients.*

(QAA 2006: 5)

When looking at the overall process of health and social care planning we therefore need to think about what will influence how we write or carry out care plans. This chapter explores some of those influences and how they affect our everyday practice of planning care. In Chapter 7 the basic quality structure of health and social care organizations is outlined in more detail, and individual and organizational accountability is discussed in more depth.

The need to be clear about how we plan care is important for a number of reasons that are often cited in policy documents and government guidelines. In general there are three main responsibilities that all of us have when carrying out practice in health and social care:

- Firstly, we are accountable to the person for whom we are providing care and we need to be able to justify our practice based on the best available evidence.

- Secondly, we are accountable to our managers and team members in delivering a good quality service to the local community.
- Thirdly, we are becoming more and more legally accountable for our practice to our professional bodies and to the government in the form of national guidelines within which we all practice. It is important to know what those laws and guidelines are but it is also just as important to be able to put them into practice every day.

These levels of responsibility will be referred to throughout this book and in each particular area of care planning. However, before we can discuss day-to-day care planning it is necessary to set the scene with some background theory.

## Levels of responsibility and a philosophy of care

A *philosophy of care* is a broad statement that will identify the purpose and theoretical underpinnings of a particular practice. It should be made visible to all who use or work within that service. Milly Smith (2004: 64) identifies a philosophy as 'the beliefs and values that shape the way each of us thinks and acts'. However, it is not only our individual philosophies that are important but how they work within the teams that we are all part of. A philosophy of care should therefore state the intention of the service and how people within it are going to go about providing such a service. In many areas of practice there will be slightly different philosophies, but you should be able to identify the basic ingredients of *purpose* and *intention* from among them. This will later be emphasized when you look at the guidance for that particular practice, which will in turn be based on evidence-based practice – i.e. research, policy, law. Social work practice, for example, is based on a set of values that all social care workers should work towards providing, including:

- *human dignity and worth* – respecting and valuing individual needs;
- *social justice* – ensuring fair access to services;
- *service to humanity* – ensuring society is taking care of its members;
- *integrity* – providing honest and accurate advice and support without judging a person or group;
- *competence* – maintaining skills and knowledge in order to provide good quality care.

### Codes of ethics

Professional organizations often provide a code of ethics (and/or practice) which will set out what a person can expect when receiving care from services provided by that organization and can be used to remove people from the professional register if not adhered to. For example, the Nursing and Midwifery Council (NMC) allows anyone to check whether a person is currently registered with the Council by simply typing in their name on the NMC online database, and all employers are expected to check that registrations are up to date. The new NMC (2008: 1) *Standards of Conduct, Performance and Ethics for Nurses and Midwives* includes the following brief guidelines:

> *The people in your care must be able to trust you with their health and well-being. To justify that trust you must:*
>
> - *Make the care of people your first concern, treating them as individuals and respecting their dignity.*
> - *Work with others to protect and promote the health and wellbeing of those in your care their families and carers and the wider community.*
> - *Provide a high standard of practice at all times.*
> - *Be open and honest, act with integrity and uphold the reputation of your profession.*

A philosophy of care should therefore outline the principles of care that a person can expect from a service and to which that service can be held accountable. Often, managers will ask for an audit of the case notes to see whether the philosophy of care is being implemented. Where there is no philosophy, guidance such as a clinical and/or social governance framework may be used or other evidence-based practice guidelines (e.g. the Single Assessment Process or SAP) (DoH 2002b). The SAP was developed from the *National Service Framework for Older People* (DoH 2001c) and is an effort to improve the quality of older people's care by taking a person-centred approach. Full details of the SAP can be obtained from the Department of Health (DoH) website. For the purpose of this book the SAP has been used as a guideline for all individual care planning as evidence of good practice and to develop the sample documentation used which can also be found in the appendix.

It is important to remember that no matter how experienced a practitioner is, there can never be enough care planning practice and there is never a perfect care plan, but we can always strive to achieve the best possible quality care for our clients and our documentation is one of the main ways of providing evidence for this. Although all documentation should remain confidential, you must be aware that if there is an incident in which practice is called into question it is your documentation that will be taken away, scrutinized and will ultimately justify the quality of your care.

## Care pathways

To help people to understand the difference between a care plan and a care pathway readers need to become familiar with this term and what it means. Care pathways are previously designed care processes that are focused on a particular disease or service provision. Their aim is to improve the quality of service provision, but rather than focusing on the person, they focus on the standard of service a person can expect to receive. Their value is therefore in the standardization of care to an acceptable level but they do not teach people *how* to plan care on an individual basis. For more information, examples and checklists on care pathways see DoH (2003d). Care pathways may already exist in your areas of practice.

> **Practice point: the philosophy of care**
>
> The philosophy of care in each individual practice area may be slightly different or more focused on one particular aspect of care. Philosophies of care are not always very evident to staff or clients although they can often be seen posted on a wall at the entrance to a building or ward. It is useful to try and find out where you can find the philosophy of care in your own workplace and hence be able to inform clients and their carers of what they can expect from your service.

## Components of a caseload audit

While we all complain about there being too much paperwork, it should be recognized why there is a need for such paperwork in the health and social care professions. Your documentation demonstrates the quality of your work and without such evidence it would be difficult to justify your professional practice. A caseload audit helps us to improve our practice by identifying flaws in the system and developing ways to improve:

> *Audit is one component of the risk management process, the aim of which is the promotion of quality. If improvements are identified and made in the processes and outcomes of healthcare, risks to the patients/clients are minimised and costs to the employer are reduced.*

(NMC 2007: 3)

The main components of what will be audited in a person's case notes are:

- general information obtained (e.g. name, date of birth, address, medication, GP, dependants);
- next of kin/lasting power of attorney/advocate;
- risk assessment (signed and dated by care coordinator and client);
- holistic assessment of need (signed and dated by care coordinator and client);
- evidence of client involvement (e.g. signature, own words used);
- crisis plan/advance statement signed and dated by care coordinator and client or advocate;
- daily record of interventions signed, dated, and designation provided;
- additional information (e.g. letter from/to GP, test results firmly secured in appropriate sections);
- a record of regular evaluation and reviews of the care plan;
- named care coordinator;
- other agencies involved identified and included in the review of the care plan with contact details recorded.

Some other basic guidelines that are transferable across all disciplines can be found in guidance on record-keeping from the NMC (2007: 2). Records should:

- be factual, consistent and accurately written in a way that the meaning is clear;
- be recorded as soon as possible after an event has occurred, providing current information on the condition of the patient/client;
- be recorded clearly and in such a way that the text cannot be erased or deleted without a record of change;
- be recorded in such a manner that any justifiable alterations or additions are dated, timed and signed or clearly attributed to a named person in an identifiable role in such a way that the original entry can still be read;
- be accurately dated, timed and signed with a signature printed alongside the first entry where this is a written record and attributed to a named person with an identifiable role where this is an electronic record;
- not include abbreviations, jargon, meaningless phrases, irrelevant speculation, offensive or subjective statements;
- be readable when photocopied or scanned;
- be recorded wherever possible with the involvement of the patient/client or their carer;
- be recorded in terms that the patient/client can understand;
- be consecutive.

Audit is therefore a quality measure that helps us to check our care plans and supporting documentation and to ensure that we adhere to a good standard of record-keeping.

## Models and theories of health and social care

The World Health Organization (WHO 1998) monitors health inequalities across the world as part of its role in improving the basic human rights of people and reducing the cost burden of ill health. However, locally, it is the role of local health and social care commissioning groups to identify local health and social care needs and provide resources to address them. This is discussed in more detail in Chapter 7. It is important to become familiar with the different models and ways of working. These can vary from organization to organization, from team to team and from individual to individual, but everyone who is involved in health and social care should be aware of their local policy guidelines and ensure that they are implemented. McKenna (1997) identifies the wide variety of interpretation of these models and theories among professionals. He suggests that there needs to be some basic definitions in order to clarify meaning:

- a *philosophy* is an overall approach to providing care that is based upon the principles of knowledge and theory;
- a *theory* is a scientifically studied concept that in most instances has been researched and can be proven;
- a *model* is a more basic or scaled down version of a theory which may or may not be based upon research;

- *a framework* is a visible process outline that can be used in everyday practice and may not be linked to a particular theory but can be used to attach to a theory or theories – i.e. a model.

Many policies that now inform our practice are based on government guidelines and models of health and social care delivery. These models fall into the following main categories (Tones 2001; Dziegielewski 2004):

- *The (bio)medical model*, which focuses on recognizing and treating signs and symptoms of disease. This model is used mainly by doctors and those working in the medical profession, especially where complex physical needs are involved.
- *The social model*, which focuses on developing the strengths and skills of individuals or groups to overcome disability and/or impairment. This model is used more widely in social care and where people suffer from a disability or long-term condition. The focus here is not upon cure but upon recovery as far as the person is able.
- *The holistic model*, which considers physical, social, psychological, spiritual and environmental needs to help the person to become more empowered over their lives. This model could be used in acute and community settings but is difficult to implement in full, given restrictions of resources and time.
- *The bio-psychosocial model*, which looks at the three main areas of people's lives (the biological, psychological and social), and attempts to incorporate a holistic approach. However this model is not truly holistic as it reduces people to three aspects of living, perhaps at the expense of others.
- *The empowerment model*, which looks at wider influences on individual health and recognizes that some of these influences may be outside the control of the individual. Encouraging adaptation to a given environment empowers and involves the person in need of care and helps them to develop skills in their own health promotion.

It could be argued from the brief outlines above that the bio-psychosocial approach is far better than the biomedical or social models and is perhaps a more realistic way of developing and planning care. However, all these models can lead to some areas of a person's life being excluded if they do not fit into a certain category. This scientific approach may ignore the whole person and the interpretation of the self by the client or patient. For example, spiritual care and what people believe in as individuals is often different from social care and the way in which groups or cultures might behave. Individual needs can therefore be ignored if we treat people simply as being part of a group (e.g. old, young, female, male etc.). It is important to remember therefore that spiritual care is not just about religion but about how a person sees themselves. This may indeed spring from religious beliefs about what it is to be human or about the personhood of the client, which can be described as how the person understands themselves through the eyes of others – for example, if a child is constantly told it is lazy by its parents the child eventually believes that it is lazy. This concept of personhood embraces spirituality and borders between psychological and social health, and is often ignored or simply overlooked. Kitwood (1997: 47) calls this 'malignant social psychology', where whole groups of people can ignore the basic human need of maintaining personhood. Greenstreet (2006) suggests that personhood is an integral part of the whole person in which spirituality connects together as a whole (see Figure 1.1).

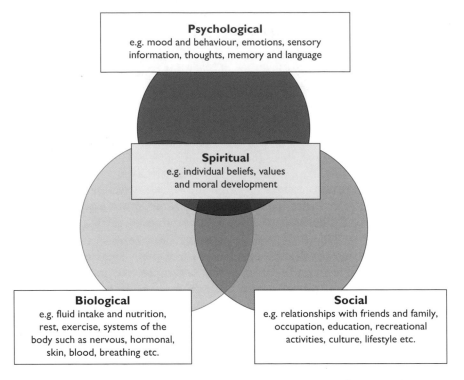

**Figure 1.1** A holistic approach to care planning

**Activity 1.1**

A classic example of how we ignore personhood can be found when a patient enters a hospital ward. Consider your own area of practice to see if any of the following apply. Patients can feel restricted in:

➡ Choosing what clothes to wear
➡ Choosing what foods to eat
➡ Choosing when to eat
➡ Choosing when to wake and when to go to sleep
➡ Choosing what personal belongings to take
➡ Choosing what name to be called

You will have seen from Activity 1.1 that it is easy to strip people of their identity and make them conform to the rules of the hospital or care home. This issue has been studied through the work of the social scientist Erving Goffman (1961) on institutionalization and does not apply just to health and social care settings but can be found in many of our institutions across the country (e.g. schools and other large organizations). Loss of personhood can lead to a loss of empowerment and control over one's health which is important to restore or enable recovery (Greenstreet 2006). A holistic model is therefore more focused on the spiritual needs of the person as well as their bio-psychosocial needs, but this approach could fail if organizational needs are not also considered. In the UK, organizations such as the NHS and social services provide the majority of care but are limited in terms of money and resources (DoH 1997). It is therefore important to recognize this limitation in balancing needs with resources and creating realistic care plans that can be delivered in practice. This care planning process at the organizational level is known as *clinical/social governance* and is discussed in more detail in Chapter 7. In addressing the difficulties encountered with other models of care planning we will therefore follow an *empowerment model* of health and social care planning that has been developed specifically for this book from the theoretical background identified above. Should you wish to find out more about the background theory to care planning, the references provided in this book will help you to explore the literature further.

## An empowerment model of health and social care planning

Empowerment seeks to help a person gain greater control over their health and social needs by taking a more holistic approach to providing support and information (Lloyd 2007). Tones (2001) suggests that an empowerment model must recognize the aspects of a person's needs shown in Figure 1.2. The shaded boxes identify where a person may be helped to have more control over their own lives, and the remaining areas are those more dependent on local and national policy. Empowering practice therefore requires a collaborative approach between the person, the practitioner and the local service providers in order to address a person's needs and access appropriate resources. Holistic or empowering practice cannot therefore be done *to* a person but rather is a theoretical or philosophical approach to working *with* people to ensure that all their needs are being met wherever possible.

In all models of health and social care delivery the consumer or client and their carer are now being encouraged to have a greater say in how their care is delivered and managed (DoH 2006b). However, the client or consumer and their carers still need to rely on the support and guidance of the practitioner who is coordinating the care, the primary health care team and the local authority to identify their needs and make appropriate provision for those needs (DoH 1997, 2001b, 2006b). The health or social care worker can play an important role as advocate for people in helping them to access the most appropriate care for their individual needs. The QAA (2006: 5) states that health and social care students/practitioners should be able to use their knowledge and skills to:

| | | |
|---|---|---|
| Health and social care public policy and law (e.g. Mental Capacity Act 2005) | **Physical needs** Life skills Health skills Self-regulatory skills | Lobbying, advocacy and mediation from local groups (e.g. voluntary organizations) |
| **Psychological needs** Reframing and adjustment of personal beliefs and attitudes | **The individual person** | **Social needs** Relationships and community empowerment, including families, teams and services |
| Social, economic and environmental issues identified and addressed (e.g. access to health and social care, public transport etc.) | **Spiritual needs** Locus of control Self-efficacy Health literacy | Critical consciousness-raising of health and social care inequalities identified from lobbying and evidence-based practice (research) |

**Figure 1.2**    An empowerment model of health and social care (adapted from Tones 2001)

- work with clients and patients to consider the range of activities that are appropriate;
- plan care and do so holistically;
- record judgements and decisions clearly.

This indicates that as practitioners we need to be able to work with individual clients to involve them in their own care needs assessment and to help them choose from the options available to them within any given health or social care environment. Sometimes, if the options are too limited or unsuitable to meet the individual person's needs, we may need to help them apply for other resources such as direct payments so that they can obtain help in meeting their needs. Direct payments are a way of helping people to become more independent of services, at the same time empowering them to take more responsibility for their own requirements. These payments are organized and monitored by local authorities and although they represent a good attempt at addressing holistic care needs and developing choice and control, they are only available for purchasing *social* care needs at this moment in time (DoH 2006a).

## Models and frameworks for care planning

The difference between 'models' and 'frameworks' is sometimes difficult to define and the terms may even be used interchangeably (McKenna 1997), but in general a *framework* is an outline or structure onto which we can attach a *model*. A robust model will be based upon theoretical and/or evidence-based practice (research). So whether we follow a medical, social, bio-psychosocial or empowerment model we will use our knowledge and skills of that model to fill out the framework of the care plan. There are some slight variations on care planning frameworks but they can be seen as being fairly similar, as shown in Table 1.1.

**Table 1.1** Care planning frameworks (adapted from Dziegielewski 2004)

| *Abbreviation* | *Process* |
| --- | --- |
| **APIE** | **Assess** current needs/problems presented upon referral/admission **Plan** goals and outcomes to address needs and increase independence/recovery **Implement** plans agreed with the client and reflect upon practice interventions/observations **Evaluate** the whole process with the multidisciplinary team and the client |
| **PIRP** | **Presenting** problem(s) upon referral/admission **Intervention** to be carried out to increase independence/recovery **Responses** to the intervention from the client **Plan** to include client responses and review interventions |
| **SOAP and SOAPIER** | **Subjective** information from referral/admission for health and social care provision **Objective** information from client (actual words) and any diagnostic tests/assessment **Assessment** of need/goals to be achieved to increase independence/recovery **Planning** interventions to address needs/goals **Implementation** of the plan in conjunction with the client and other agencies **Evaluation** of the care planning process **Response** of the client to the process |
| **DAP and DAPE** | **Data** gathered upon referral/admission **Assessment** of the client's needs/problems **Planning** to address client's needs/problems and increase independence/recovery **Evaluation** and education – information provided in meeting the above needs |

For the purpose of this book we will be using the APIE framework because it is a very familiar one to many people in health and social care practice and the stages help us to identify what needs to be achieved quickly and efficiently. The APIE framework is divided into four stages, as shown in Figure 1.3.

The stages flow into each other rather than following a linear pathway so it is important to recognize that care planning can be a 'spiral' process with many twists and turns throughout the course of a person's care plan. You may need to focus a lot

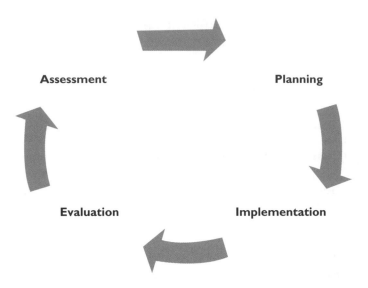

**Assessment**          **Planning**

**Evaluation**          **Implementation**

**Figure 1.3**   The APIE framework for care planning

of attention on the assessment stage at first, but all the other stages are just as important for the care plan to work. Many health and social care textbooks focus on the assessment stage and will help you to identify a person's individual needs; however, this is a rather useless exercise if you do not know how to follow the rest of the framework. You may find that as things develop you will need to change the care plan at short notice or re-assess a particular area of care.

The model used in this book to build on the APIE framework is the *empowerment model*, which helps us to stay focused on the needs of the individual as well as the needs of the organization.

---

**Activity 1.2**

How many assessment tools are used in your area of practice and how many of those are you familiar with? You will need to discuss your findings with a mentor or manager. Some assessment tools require training which you may identify as a need for your own continual professional development (CPD).

---

A multi-professional approach

In many health and social policy texts the World Health Organization's (1978: 1) *Declaration of Alma-Ata*, USSR is often cited as providing an agreed definition of health, which includes a whole-person or holistic approach to care as: 'a state of complete physical, mental and social well-being and not merely the absence of disease or infirmity'.

This indicates that practitioners should not focus purely upon illness or disability but on the strengths of individual people and their environments. Many models for care provision are now following a multidisciplinary/multi-professional route to avoid duplication and to improve communication between services.

## Components of a care plan

The care planning process consists of at least five pieces of documentation:

- The *initial assessment* to gather basic information such as contact details of the person, their relatives and their doctor, any known allergies/conditions and medications taken.
- A *holistic or bio-psychosocial assessment* which seeks more in-depth information on the person's needs.
- A *risk assessment* to identify need and prioritize risk.
- A *care plan* which outlines *needs* identifies *plans or goals* to address those needs, *implements* certain actions to achieve those goals and *evaluates* the whole process. The care plan is devised using a SMART approach: *specific, measurable, achievable, realistic* and *timely*. This acronym helps us to remember how to write a care plan and will be discussed in more detail in Chapter 3.
- A *record sheet* to document activities in relation to the care plan and as evidence for the evaluation stage.

These are the documents we will be using to complete a care plan for a fictitious client called Brian throughout the rest of this book. (They are also available in the appendix for photocopying.) Remember that these documents are for practise purposes *only* and you will need to make sure that you use the appropriate documentation for your area of practice. However, documents of this type all tend to follow a similar outline.

**Example of initial assessment documentation**

| | |
|---|---|
| Completed by ................................................ Date ........................ | |
| 1. Name of person being assessed | Address |
| Date of birth | Telephone number(s) |
| 2. Name of GP | Address of general practitioner |
| | Telephone number of general practitioner |

| 3. Name of next of kin | Address of next of kin |
|---|---|
| | Telephone numbers(s) |
| 4. Marital status<br>Married       Single<br>Divorced       Civil partnership<br>Other ...................................... | 5. Religion |
| 6. Medication currently being taken (*add separate sheet if necessary*) | 7. Disabilities or impairments (*e.g. wears glasses, uses a hearing aid etc.*) |
| 8. Any known allergies? | 9. Dietary requirements |
| 10. Any dependants (*e.g. children, elderly parents etc.*)? | 11. Other agencies involved (*e.g. social worker, probation etc.*) |
| Contact details of dependants | Contact details of other agencies involved |
| 12. Current or previous occupation | 13. Any other requirements/urgent needs (*e.g. diabetes, epilepsy*) |

## Personal assessment

| Assessment information | Observations (please complete all boxes to show that they have been addressed) |
|---|---|
| **Biological: do you have any needs in the following areas?** | **Please state in the person's own words where possible and record any measurements (including frequency where required)** |
| Breathing | |

| | |
|---|---|
| Eating (including appetite) and food preparation | |
| Sleeping and rest | |
| Washing and bathing | |
| Dressing | |
| Moving and walking | |
| Exercise and activities | |
| Hygiene and self-care (*e.g. hair, nails, teeth, using the toilet, skin care etc.*) | |
| Maintaining/losing weight | |
| Vital signs: blood pressure, temperature, pulse, skin colour and texture | |
| **Psychological: do you have any needs in the following areas?** | |
| Memory | |
| Thought disturbances | |
| Moods and emotions | |

| | |
|---|---|
| Beliefs about others | |
| Perceptions | |
| Sensations (*e.g. taste, touch, smell, sight and sound*) | |
| **Social: do you have any needs in the following areas?** | |
| Family support | |
| Friends/peer support | |
| Meaningful occupation (*including work, hobbies etc.*) | |
| Group membership | |
| Recreational activities | |
| Significant relationships | |
| **Spiritual: do you have any needs in the following areas?** | |
| Personal religious beliefs | |
| Personal cultural beliefs | |

## General risk assessment    *Diagnosis*

| Area of risk | Current needs | Positive risks taken |
|---|---|---|
| Hypothermia | | |
| Neglect | | |
| Abuse, physical, emotional, financial | | |
| Exploitation | | |
| Slips, trips and falls | | |
| Isolation | | |
| Nutrition and hydration | | |
| Suicide/self-harm | | |
| Violence/aggression | | |

**Care plan using the SMART formula** (if only using one sheet remember to number needs in order of priority)

| Patient name | | Date of birth | |
|---|---|---|---|
| **Needs** (*Specific: in person's own words where possible*) | **Goals** (*Measurable and achievable: including any assessment tool measurements*) | **Interventions** (*Realistic*) | **Evaluation** (*Timely*) |
| | | | |
| **Signatures** | Care coordinator | Client | Date |

**Daily record sheet: to be completed by care coordinator or by designated person and countersigned by care coordinator**

| Date | Record to be made at least once daily or on every contact | Signature and designation |
|---|---|---|
| | | |

An empowerment model of care planning must consider the needs of the individual and the resources available to meet those needs. It is ineffective not to consider these two basic components in equal weighting. Focusing on one area of need without identifying the resources available to meet that need can lead to failure in the care plan before you even begin. The constant balancing act between resources and needs can be addressed through regular contact with your colleagues and by working as a team towards meeting individual needs (see Chapter 3 for more information on working in a multidisciplinary team). Often needs and resources are diverse and some creativity may be required in matching them up. This is the skill of an experienced practitioner which we all have to learn, sometimes through trial and error or by taking *positive* risks. The process involves a constant awareness of being *person-centred*, identifying *diverse needs* or skills and *team working* towards achieving specified individual goals. Consider the following hot topic before we go on to explore these ideas in more detail.

---

### Hot topic

There will be legal and ethical implications when we identify that we cannot meet particular individual needs. How might we overcome this problem and what laws might be used to ensure the needs of our clients are met? You are not expected to know every law available but you should be familiar with some of the laws in everyday use in your own areas of practice (e.g. The Mental Health Act, The Mental Capacity Act, The Human Rights Act etc.).

---

## Taking a person-centred approach

The empowerment model should always centre on individual needs, paying full attention to biological, psychological, sociological and spiritual needs to maintain personhood (Kitwood 1997; Greenstreet 2006). This requires a flexible approach so that we do not try to slot people into particular categories. Each person is unique in their skills and abilities and it is our responsibility to help them use those abilities to aid their recovery. Wherever possible people should be encouraged to make their own decisions based on the best available evidence we can present to them. However, they also have the right to make the wrong decision (under the Mental Capacity Act 2005) and we should not deny our help to them if they do. Too many people are denied services because they do not fit into a particular category or label within our organizations. It is well worth remembering the five principles of the Mental Capacity Act 2005 when planning individualized care:

❶ Every adult has the right to make his or her own decisions and must be assumed to have capacity to make them unless it is proved otherwise.
❷ A person must be given all practicable help before anyone treats them as not being able to make their own decisions.
❸ Just because an individual makes what might be seen as an unwise decision, they should not be treated as lacking capacity to make that decision.
❹ Anything done or any decision made on behalf of a person who lacks capacity must be done in their best interests.

⑤ Anything done for or on behalf of a person who lacks capacity should be the least restrictive of their basic rights and freedoms.

## Recognizing strengths and respecting diversity

An empowerment model can only work by recognizing strengths and respecting individual diversity (Lloyd 2009). In order to be empowered, a person must feel in control of their own destiny within their particular spiritual and sociological environment. When we take someone out of their familiar environment we weaken them by taking away their resources. This is why it is important to help people stay as close to their own homes as possible and in a safe and comfortable environment. This will be discussed in more detail in Chapters 3 and 4. Diverse skills within a team of practitioners should also be identified and matched with the needs of the individual person. In this way, the best care can be provided using the skills of the most appropriate practitioner for that person. The DoH (2008a) has refocused the care programme approach to be more person-centred by recognizing individual needs and strengths. This approach requires that there is more choice and more options for people to choose from rather than a standard approach to care planning. It can be very difficult therefore in practice to ensure that individual needs, strengths and wishes have been addressed without some model to remind us.

## Working in partnership with individuals and teams towards common goals

An empowerment model requires that all members of the health and social care team work together to ensure that good quality care is provided according to their clinical and social governance agendas (see Chapter 7 for more information on clinical and social governance). This includes ensuring that the patient or client features strongly throughout the whole process (Lloyd 2009). This is not a sole venture but requires the support or 'reciprocal determinism' (Tones 2001: 7) of family, friends, other professionals and resources. This is discussed in more detail in Chapter 6, but requires maintaining the individual person at the centre of the process and then using our resources, knowledge and skills to support them. Figure 1.4 outlines the whole care planning framework with the empowerment model attached.

As can be seen in Figure 1.4, the whole person and their support system must remain at the centre of care planning. The different stages require the practitioner to take different approaches to providing care that most suits the individual at the centre of the care plan. All of the stages are just as important as each other and each stage requires different skills. The main four stages of care planning each have their own unique contribution to the process that if not addressed will contribute to poor quality care being provided. The following points outline the main practice areas of each stage.

● *Assessment* is mentioned in all the policy documents as a right of most individuals and their carers in need. This can be carried out using assessment tools to produce an in-depth analysis of the person's need. Assessment requires good communication

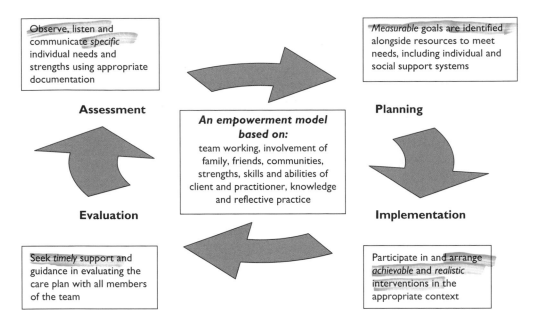

**Figure 1.4** The complete care planning process, centred on empowerment

skills and the ability to observe physical, social and psychological changes. The appropriate documentation must be used and must be available as evidence of involvement.

- *Planning* requires the ability to identify goals with the person in need and offer a choice of approaches or interventions to address those goals. Goals can be short- or long-term but it is important that they are written in a way that the individual person understands. They should also be carried out as close to home as possible using the strengths and supports that are already familiar and available to the person.

- *Implementation* of the care plan requires identifying ways to achieve goals that will demonstrate to the person (and our managers) that the health and social care provided will lead to recovery for the individual. These outcomes should be measurable and focused on individual need, so may involve some positive risk-taking.

- *Evaluation* is the stage where the whole care plan is reviewed formally with the team who are contributing to the delivery of health and social care. This may be only one or two people in less complex cases. The evaluation stage reminds us that we must re-assess the person's needs at regular intervals to ensure that the current care plan is still required and to identify any changes that have taken place in the meantime. If we do not evaluate our care formally we may not notice subtle changes that take place over a period of time that can indicate recovery, however small. The opportunity to discuss the overall care plan during supervision is necessary to help us find our blind spots or to find alternative ways of supporting the client.

The following chapters will look in more detail at each stage of the care planning process and will identify the skills and knowledge that will help you to provide person-centred care for an individual.

---

**Activity 1.3**

Before moving on to the next chapter, take some time to explore current care planning practices in your own area of work.

 Are there many different types of care planning taking place or is there one main care plan that all practitioners work to?

 How involved is the person in creating their own care plan and how would you know this?

---

## Chapter summary

➡ Models and frameworks help us to use knowledge and skills in practice.
➡ Care planning needs to be aware of a whole-system approach.
➡ An empowerment model helps us to keep the individual at the centre of the process.
➡ The care planning process is a continuous one of assessment and evaluation in practice.

---

## Self-assessment questions

 Why do we need a framework to outline the process?

 What are the five main components of the care planning documentation?

 Why is it important to maintain personhood during care planning?

 Identify the four main areas of a basic care plan.

# 2 The assessment of needs

**This chapter will help you to:**

➡ Outline the assessment stage of the care planning process.
➡ Identify barriers to effective assessment.
➡ Focus on the individual person's needs.
➡ Explore the therapeutic relationship.

## Introduction

*Personalising services means making services fit for everyone's needs not just for those of the people who make the loudest demands. When they need it, all patients want care that is personal to them.*

(DoH 2008b: 3)

The previous chapter examined how assessment fits within the overall care planning process, and this chapter will identify the skills needed for carrying out effective assessments, as a foundation for ensuring high standards of planning and care. It is at this stage that the care planning process most often begins and maintains good quality care, so it is important to be aware of how this stage fits into the rest of the care planning process. Assessment of needs can be of a particular group for service development purposes, or of an individual's needs. It is important to be clear that while knowledge of care or service provision is useful for accessing resources, the majority of this book will focus on care planning for the *individual* client. However, many of the skills you will use or learn as assessment tools will help you plan services on a wider scale and so will be useful in numerous contexts. This chapter will help you to explore this crucial stage more thoroughly and identify areas of practice that might help or prevent a good assessment taking place.

## What is assessment?

In health and social care services, assessment is the term used to define the process of observation and enquiry by which the practitioner and the multidisciplinary team get to know the person and their individual needs. Assessment therefore identifies how the person's physical, psychological, social and spiritual needs are being addressed (or not) and what areas need to be addressed. However, when things go wrong in practice there is often a systematic or process breakdown which may be the result of the assessment area of practice not being addressed in enough depth. In the inquiry in to the death of Victoria Climbié, the DoH (2003a: 7) stated that:

> Appropriate assessment lies at the heart of effective service delivery for a whole range of health and social care provision. Its purpose is to identify and evaluate individuals' presenting needs and how they constrain or support his/her capacity to live a full and independent life. Councils should ensure that individuals are active partners in the assessment of their needs. Appropriate service provision can then be planned both in the immediate and in the longer term to promote or preserve independence.

The previous chapter identified a framework for care planning that can help us to build a model of care that is evidence-based and focused on the individual in need of health and/or social care. We will now take each stage of the care planning process and look at them in more detail in the next four chapters. This will help us to identify how each stage is different and yet at the same time linked. Figure 2.1, first introduced in Chapter 1, will be completed as we go through each stage, helping you to identify the important differences. Along with being the starting point, assessment will very often be the mid-point and the end-point too. It will also be demonstrated during this process how we can keep the individual involved and at the centre of the care plan while building our observations and skills around them.

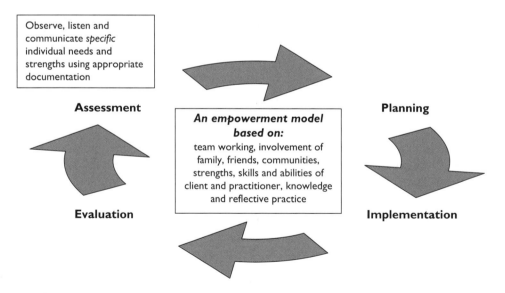

**Figure 2.1** The care planning process using the APIE framework: assessment stage

In Chapter 1 an empowerment model was identified to help us remember the three core activities of good quality care which were:

- person-centred;
- identifying strengths and diversity;
- team working.

This approach is supported by the White Paper *Our Health, Our Care, Our Say* (DoH 2006a) that gathered information on health and social care reform in the community from a wide variety of participants and identified the three following principles:

- *Putting people more in control over their health and care* by providing more information (health literacy) and supporting them in making decisions and taking risks. This includes gaining access to the right information that is person-centred.
- *Enabling and supporting health independence and well-being* by recognizing individual and cultural differences and working with the person within these boundaries. Such diverse practice will be necessary to maintain a person-centred approach and to address individual needs.
- *Rapid and convenient access to high quality and convenient care* by becoming aware of what the other members of your team can do and how to access local services quickly and efficiently.

These wider areas of practice can be remembered using the following list of key words involved in an empowering assessment and care planning process:

- *advocacy* by helping people to identify and address their own needs;
- *access* in ensuring that individual differences are recognized and accommodated,
- *action* by encouraging relationships and routes for *advocacy* and *access* to develop.

The above areas should be taken into account from the very first assessment interview and be visible throughout the care plan in maintaining personhood and individualized care planning. The initial assessment will gather much of the information that we need to start putting an empowerment model of care planning into practice and should be recorded as soon as possible. We will now look at how to carry out this stage in more detail as we gather information from our case study patient, Brian.

## Introducing Brian

Throughout this book, reference will be made to a fictitious person named Brian who will be discussed in each chapter in relation to his health and social care needs. Brian is a single man living alone with a long-term condition that most of us are familiar with – diabetes. He has managed his condition himself for most of his life but is now asking for some help to get it back under control. His condition will not be discussed in any great detail here as the purpose of introducing Brian is to help us make the care planning process more realistic. Brian therefore could be any person that you are helping at this moment in time. The important area of practice to remember is that whoever you are planning care with, they remain at the centre of the process. This is known as a case study approach because it follows one particular person (or group) through a process.

> Brian is a 55-year-old man who lives alone in an isolated village. He has suffered from diabetes all his life but has managed to take care of his own needs with regular medication and support from his GP. Brian worked in a factory for most of his life but when his mobility became poor he had to give up work and took early retirement 12 months ago. He also had to give up his car because he could no longer afford to keep it on as he is now living on a pension. Brian has never married and has no children but his older brother, Bill, lives in the next town and he is in regular contact with him and his family by telephone, which is an important lifeline to Brian. Brian also spends Christmas and birthdays with his brother. Brian's brother has two sons but they both live and work away from home. Brian used to like going to local football matches and visiting the village pub, although he does not drink alcohol because of his diabetes. Brian is becoming very concerned about his diabetes and his general quality of life. His pension restricts his ability to buy the right food for his diabetes and he has noticed that he is getting more irregular readings when he uses his blood sugar monitoring kit. Up until now he has been able to manage his diabetes with very little support from anyone and has led an independent life so he cannot understand why it has suddenly become so unstable.

> **Practice point: providing holistic care**
>
> Consider the models of health and social care identified in Chapter 1 and think about which one is more evident in your area of work. This will help you to see how models can influence what we might do next for Brian. Would you send him to another service saying that you cannot meet his needs or would you help him to identify his needs and access the resources he needs? Is your organization service-led or focused on person-centred care?

## Initial assessment

This is a pre-assessment stage where you will need to gather all the basic information. It is very important to gather this information as it may need to be used in an emergency or when an appointment needs to be changed. It will therefore need to be checked regularly so that updated information can be added. This is particularly important in an emergency and for that reason this information should be kept at the very front of a person's case notes.

**Example of initial assessment documentation**

| Completed by | |
|---|---|
| A.N. Other (RN)..............................................Date ...01/01/2010.............. | |
| 1. Name of person being assessed<br><br>Brian David Jones | Address<br><br>44 The Avenue, Somewhere Village, Nr Hometown, Homeshire H11 2LL |
| Date of birth<br><br>      01/01/1955 | Telephone number(s)<br><br>      01790 666666 |
| 2. Name of general practitioner<br><br>Dr J Evans | Address of general practitioner<br><br>The Practice, High Street, Hometown H11 3LL |
| | Telephone number(s) of general practitioner<br><br>01790 445544<br>01790 554455 out of hours |
| 3. Name of next of kin<br><br>Mr William John Jones | Address of next of kin<br><br>24 The Street, Hometown, Homeshire H11 4LL |
| | Telephone number(s)<br><br>01790 665566 |
| 4. Marital status<br><br>Married         Single √<br>Divorced       Civil partnership<br>Other ..................................... | 5. Religion<br><br>Chapel |
| 6. Medication currently being taken (*add separate sheet if necessary*)<br><br>Insulin | 7. Disabilities or impairments (*e.g. wears glasses, uses a hearing aid etc.*)<br><br>Prescription glasses |
| 8. Any known allergies?<br><br>None known to Brian | 9. Dietary requirements<br><br>Vegetarian and diabetic |
| 10. Any dependants (*e.g. children, elderly parents etc.*)?<br><br>No | 11. Other agencies involved (*e.g. social worker, probation etc.*)<br><br>No |

| Contact details of dependants | Contact details of other agencies involved |
|---|---|
| None | None known |
| 12. Current or previous occupation | 13. Any other requirements/urgent needs (*e.g. diabetes, epilepsy*) |
| Factory worker for 35 years – retired 12 months ago | Carries insulin pen at all times |

As you can see from the completed initial assessment sheet, all the boxes must be completed so that other professionals examining the form at a later date can be sure that every question was asked.

## Assessment of the environment: improving access to services

Although advocacy for Brian is our main goal there are often factors that can get in the way of this happening despite our good intentions. This can lead to burnout which causes staff to give up trying before they have even begun. Therefore, before you begin to carry out a fuller assessment with Brian you will need to prepare yourself and the environment so that you can gather as much information in one meeting as possible. There are many factors that can get in the way of a successful assessment, such as shortage of time or enough staff, noise or lack of privacy. As practitioners we should be thinking all the time about how we can improve *access* to services so that the process becomes more open to the needs of the people we work with. Try out Activity 2.1.

---

**Activity 2.1**

Consider the following locations and how easy or otherwise it might be to carry out a successful assessment in each of them. How would you improve the environment in each?

➡ A care home for older people
➡ A busy medical ward
➡ A school for children with behavioural and/or learning difficulties
➡ A job club for adults with mental health problems
➡ A secure environment such as a prison, police station or locked ward
➡ A person's own home

---

Many environments are difficult to change in structure although for health and safety reasons if nothing else we should always be aware of the implications of the environments in which we work. Small changes can often be made to allow us to spend more time with a client so that a proper assessment can take place. Freeing up time and space is everyone's responsibility so that we can spend that time providing a good quality service for which a full and proper assessment is essential.

## Practitioner access and barriers to assessment

While all practitioners must attempt to carry out an assessment that is fair and non-judgemental in accordance with their own codes of professional conduct, there may also be aspects of their own practice that become barriers to an effective assessment. The important issue here is to have an awareness of access and barriers to effective working, and the confidence that you have done all you can to address them. If there are barriers that may prevent an assessment then the practitioner has a duty to notify their managers and colleagues of these barriers so that they may be taken into consideration when planning care. Barriers may include:

- language and culture;
- time and resources;
- skills and knowledge;
- values and attitudes;
- gender and respect.

It would probably be considered unethical practice if a practitioner were to attempt to carry out an assessment without considering potential barriers to a successful outcome and may even be regarded as neglect if some of the above issues are overlooked. The Mental Capacity Act 2005 has made it a criminal offence to neglect the needs of people who may not be able to seek help by themselves. Therefore, the values and attitudes of practitioners towards the person they are assessing should at all times be respectful of their individual needs. The DoH guidance on *Refocusing the Care Programme Approach* in mental health care (2008a: 7) provides a statement of values and attitudes for practitioners which includes:

- respecting and recognizing the individual as a person first and a patient second;
- supporting individual and diverse roles in all areas of life including spirituality, leisure, family, education, occupation, housing, creativity, self-management and self-nurture;
- encouraging independence and self-determination;
- carers being recognized and supported;
- services organized based on therapeutic partnerships and relationships that require good listening, sharing, understanding, organizing and communicating skills;
- the care planning process should be based on long-term engagement requiring trust, team working and commitment.

There are other barriers to effective communication, and consequently assessment, that have been highlighted in the policy document *Essence of Care* (DoH 2003c):

- lack of space or a quite room – often occurs in hospital or busy office settings;
- lack of time  – you will need to allow as much time as possible; saying 'I've got five minutes' hardly communicates a willingness to listen;

- lack of resources (e.g. pen, paper, assessment tools, table, comfortable chairs);
- distractions by others, noise, a television or telephone;
- pain and discomfort;
- lack of communication and/or assessment skills.

There are many areas when attempting to make a full assessment that, unless identified, may affect the quality of the care planning process from the very beginning. It is important to recognize as soon as possible what might get in the way, at which point you can think about how you are going to address the problem. Making sure that we get as much information as possible from Brian will require good communication skills which can then be developed as part of the therapeutic relationship.

## Developing the therapeutic relationship

Although we should all be as professional as possible when carrying out an assessment it is important to be warm and friendly at the same time. This will develop trust and encourage the client to be open and honest about their needs. If they think that you are going to judge them or, worse, criticize their actions, they are unlikely to tell you what is bothering them (Berreta 2003). Watson and West (2006: 44) state that, 'to work in partnership and empower clients it is important to communicate with them in a way that those using the service can understand and can build upon'. They go on to identify four means of communication:

- *verbal* – what is said and discussed using words and language that are recognizable to everyone involved;
- *non-verbal* – gestures and mannerisms have a vocabulary that is culturally determined: clothes and hairstyles communicate information as do positioning, eye contact and posture;
- *para-verbal* – interjections of sounds or words such as 'uh huh' to indicate that we are following the conversation. This can become distracting if over-used;
- *written* – documentation of the discussions held and recorded in a way that is clear and concise.

---

**Activity 2.2**

Consider whether in your own practice you are aware of the following unspoken or non-verbal interactions in your everyday practice.

➡ Being empathic by listening to and trying to understand what the person has to say

➡ Being genuine by focusing completely on what you are doing and how it makes you feel

➡ Being caring towards the person, not trying to hurry them or dismiss what they have to say

The above skills are all quite hard to develop to any level but experience will help you in this. These skills are known as the core components of a therapeutic relationship, as developed by Carl Rogers (1967), a well-known counsellor who pioneered the person-centred approach. He suggested that in order to be empathic and genuine we must accept the person without judgement and focus on what they have to say. By helping the person to do this, perhaps for the first time in their life, you will be rewarded with information that they may not have told anyone before. Being empathic and genuine therefore requires good communication and questioning skills that are *observable*. The practitioner needs to demonstrate compassion and an understanding of their client's suffering. A recent report by the King's Fund (Firth-Cozens and Cornwell 2009: 3) suggests that compassionate care is not always evident in health and social care. The authors quote a carer they interviewed as part of their research who had experienced poor quality care when accompanying her terminally ill husband to hospital. Her husband was then listened to holistically by a doctor in a hospice: 'She spent all the time he needed, she answered his questions honestly, she allowed silence and she addressed the whole man, the one he was as well as the one he had become'.

## Basic communication skills and values required to carry out an assessment

The following skills and values will be developed as we become experienced in the care planning process. The important thing to remember here is to not get so concerned about your communication skills that you do not allow the person to tell their whole story (Kleinman 1988).

- *Honesty* – say if you do not understand what is meant. Ask questions. This demonstrates that you are listening, but be careful not to *direct* the person by asking closed or leading questions. Such questions limit the answer that could be given (e.g. 'Have you been out Brian?' The answer may be no, but if you ask, 'What have you been doing with yourself since I saw you last?' Brian may offer more information).
- *Openness* – your non-verbal communication will give you away if you are not open with the person about what you think and feel. Sometimes this will encourage further explanation by demonstrating that you are paying attention and waiting to hear what they have to say, but be careful not to fall into a sympathetic mode which may be counter-productive. For example, saying, 'Oh my goodness, that must have been terrible, I don't know how you coped,' indicates your own distress and may prevent the person telling you more. Likewise adopting a closed posture does not convey that you are open or even interested in what the person has to say.
- *Attending* – this requires 'listening' with your ears *and* your eyes in order to detect changes of tone, speech and non-verbal behaviour, and even body temperature and colour. Just as the person will notice a change in your behaviour, you should also attend to their behaviour the whole time you are with them (Berreta 2003). If they are becoming agitated or upset you will know that you need to respond by giving some para-verbal reactions such as 'mmmmm', or 'uh huh' or simply by nodding

your head. This demonstrates that you are listening to them, but be careful that you do not overdo it in your eagerness as it can become quite annoying, especially during silences. Silences are opportunities for people to gather their thoughts and think about what they want to say, and the client may begin to feel rushed if you keep trying to encourage them with your para-verbal responses.

- *Guiding* – the above approaches are basic skills only and there are many books available on communication skills in general. However, if we are taking a person-centred approach we should remember to open and close all our conversations within the appropriate cultural traditions in which we practice. These include introducing ourselves and our purpose for meeting appropriately, asking the person we are meeting what they would like to be called and ending the conversation with how the information will be taken forward, or what will happen next (see Chapter 4 for more discussion on cultural diversity).

When you first meet Brian it is because his diabetes is unstable and he needs some support with getting it back on track. However, as you get to know Brian you will find out more things about him that will inform you about how to plan his care together. Although there are various assessment tools available to assess needs your most important tools are your eyes and your ears. Your observation skills will become attuned to Brian the more you get to know him, but at first you will have to learn to tune yourself into what makes Brian a unique individual. You will be looking and listening for signs that his health and social care needs are being met using the above communication skills and values.

---

**Practice point: observing communication skills in action**

Before moving on, take some time to observe your colleagues in practice for the above basic skills (even if it is only on the telephone). You may notice that skilled practitioners are identifiable by their ability to develop and use their communication skills without it being that evident (or mechanistic) to other people. Until you start to watch them in practice you may not notice the subtle ways in which they extract information from people, while at the same time appearing to have a general conversation about everyday events such as the weather, the garden or sport.

---

Once we have listened to all that Brian has to say to us we can complete the first main assessment stage. As Brian is a fictitious character we will need to assume some of this information but in practice remember that you should clarify and ask questions about anything that you are not sure of.

## Personal assessment

| | Observations (please complete all boxes to show that they have been addressed) |
|---|---|
| **Biological: do you have any needs in the following areas?** | **Please state in the person's own words where possible and record any measurements (including frequency where required)** |
| Breathing | No |
| Eating (including appetite) and food preparation | Cannot always obtain the right food for my diabetes<br>Cannot be bothered to prepare food sometimes<br>Eating too many carbohydrates |
| Sleeping and rest | I am sleeping a lot of the time |
| Washing and bathing | I can manage this by myself |
| Dressing | Sometimes doing up laces is a struggle |
| Moving and walking | I have pain a lot when walking |
| Exercise and activities | Very limited because of pain in my legs |
| Hygiene and self-care (*e.g. hair, nails, teeth, using the toilet, skin care etc.*) | No |
| Maintaining/losing weight | Am probably overweight: 5ft 5 and 13 stone |
| Vital signs: blood pressure, temperature, pulse, skin colour and texture | Blood pressure raised 140/90 |
| **Psychological: do you have any needs in the following areas?** | |
| Memory | No |
| Thought disturbances | No |

| Moods and emotions | Get black moods sometimes |
|---|---|
| Beliefs about others | No |
| Perceptions | No |
| Sensations (*e.g. taste, touch, smell, sight and sound*) | No |
| **Social: do you have any needs in the following areas?** | |
| Family support | My brother but he cannot help much |
| Friends/peer support | No friends now I've left work |
| Meaningful occupation (*including work, hobbies etc.*) | Bored a lot of the time |
| Group membership | Not a member of any |
| Recreational activities | Used to visit the pub and watch local football team |
| Significant relationships | Have none |
| **Spiritual: do you have any needs in the following areas?** | |
| Personal religious beliefs | Chapel but have not been for some time – I miss it now |
| Personal cultural beliefs | Villagers want to know your business so keep to myself<br>I am not much use to myself or anyone else now that I have given up work |

## General risk assessment

| Area of risk | Current needs | Positive risks taken |
|---|---|---|
| Hypothermia | No | |
| Neglect | Diet sometimes neglected | Brother helps me sometimes |
| Abuse | No | |
| Exploitation | No | |
| Slips, trips and falls | Pain in legs sometimes makes me fall | Use furniture in house and walking stick outside |
| Isolation | Retired so not very sociable | None |
| Nutrition and hydration | Sometimes eat wrong foods for diabetes | Talk to doctor about it sometimes |
| Suicide/self-harm | Wonder what's the point sometimes | Not good at talking to people |
| Violence/aggression | No | |

**Activity 2.3**

Consider the following diagram again. With regard to Brian, what areas will you be observing for his health and social care needs and strengths?

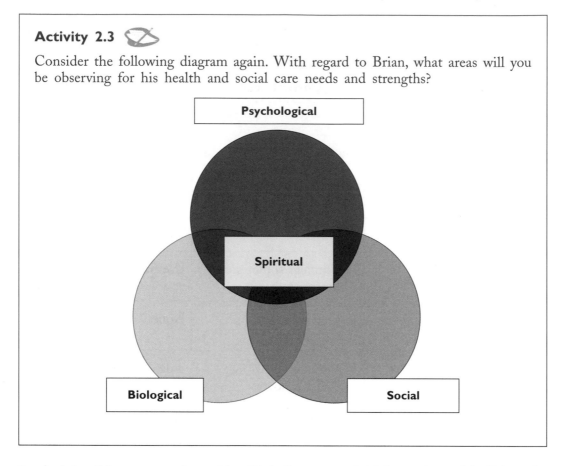

In Activity 2.3 you may have identified from your initial meeting with Brian the following areas of concern:

- *Biological* – Brian suffers from *diabetes* and is a *vegetarian*. These two aspects of his diet could have a detrimental effect on each other and may need further exploration. Brian also wears prescription glasses which indicates that his *eyesight* may be poor. He also has *mobility* problems which will affect his ability to manage his health care needs and obtain the appropriate resources.
- *Psychological* – Brian no longer works and is quite *isolated* at home in a village environment. He may be at a *loss* about what to do with himself and his *sense of purpose* now that he is not occupied in paid work. Brian's diabetes has caused some impairment to his mobility and general health care which may affect his *mood* if he feels that he has no control over what is happening to him.

- *Sociological* – Brian may have lost *contact* with many of his friends from work. It is not clear if he still visits the pub or goes to chapel at this stage. Brian may feel that he has no interests that will help him to socialize with other people. He has some contact with his *brother* Bill who lives in the next town but due to his mobility problems he has difficulty getting there and to see his GP. As Brian has recently given up his car it is unlikely that he has used *public transport* for many years.
- *Spiritual* – Brian is a member of the local *chapel* but we need to find out if he still attends and whether he finds this supportive and empowering. Brian may not know how to occupy himself and develop his *strengths* since finishing work. He may need to re-evaluate his personal *beliefs* about work and leisure and develop more skills in *meaningful* activities that could be a creative outlet for him (e.g. art).

The important thing at this stage is to ensure that you have identified *all* of Brian's needs. Later on in the process there may be cause to explore some of those needs in more detail and you may require specialist services to achieve that. This stage is about *identification of needs*, not *addressing them immediately* as you may need to go away and find out some more information on what help is available. This is where it is important not to get too caught up in your own needs and whether you can help this client with all aspects of their care. Do not worry that you do not have all the answers: the main concern is that you know how to find out and are not afraid to ask. Many professional codes of practice say that this is a requirement of practitioners in health and social care and that you must report to your managers anything that you do not feel competent to do (e.g. NMC 2008).

## Involving people in their care plan: advocacy

There is growing evidence that people want and need to be more involved in the care planning process and it is no more evident than in inquiry documents that have been produced following an investigation into practices which could and should have been more person-centred (Green 2007). Such lapses often occur on occasions when it is difficult to involve a person in their care. This may be because they are very ill, unconscious, too distressed or very young or old. Working with vulnerable people allows us all to become at risk of failing to meet the needs of certain individuals either through a lack of respect, knowledge or skills. It is not always the case that people are deliberately harmful to one another but that they do in fact believe they are doing the right thing for that person. It is only by acting upon and communicating our practice and our knowledge that we are able to make sense of practice and where necessary improve it (Ghaye 2000; Hawkins and Shohet 2006). The following list will help you to think about how to involve a person more in their assessment and care plan.

- Do allow enough time to gather all the necessary information.
- Do listen carefully to what the person has to say.
- Do allow silences so the person can gather their thoughts.
- Do pay attention in order to demonstrate that you care about what they have to say.

- Don't rush the person by ending their sentences.
- Don't give non-verbal information that you are bored, tired or impatient.
- Don't forget to document as soon as possible.
- Don't be afraid to seek help/information if you need it.

In many areas of practice things can go right or wrong depending upon how much knowledge we have of the people we work with and the resources, skills and barriers to meeting their health and social care needs. You may have begun to recognize by now that care planning is not an exact science but a skill or even an art, involving matching individual needs with the resources and skills available to you. However, there are times (which are thankfully quite rare) when things go terribly wrong. It is often not the case that it is a deliberate act on behalf of staff but more likely an oversight or lack of knowledge and/or information that has led to tragic consequences. It would however be neglectful of us not to discuss those here so that we can be aware of the possible areas of practice in which things can go wrong. By developing our awareness we can help to prevent such things happening in the future.

## When practice is not always effective

It has already been identified that neglectful practices should not be tolerated at anyone's expense. The Mental Capacity Act 2005 is not just for people who lack capacity but exists to ensure everyone's basic human rights and consequently that their needs are being met. Chapter 3 will discuss in more detail how personhood can often be neglected, a situation which Kitwood (1997) terms 'malignant social psychology' and which is also known as 'malignant alienation' (Watts and Morgan 1994). A critical account of the 'unpopular patient' has also been given by Felicity Stockwell (1972) who identified that people were likely to be more unpopular if they were of a different age or cultural background to their carers and/or if they suffered from an illness that made communication difficult. The person's length of stay in a hospital bed was also detrimental to their care unless it was being provided by people who were not prejudiced towards them.

The causes of alienation, prejudice and unpopularity may therefore be due to a number of factors but should be identified and addressed as soon as possible to prevent further harm. The following are some common areas that need to be explored with the client as soon as it becomes evident that they are agitated or upset, which could lead to communication difficulties and alienation.

- *Pain* can cause many of us to be irritable but it is difficult for anyone to judge what constitutes pain and sometimes there may be no reason for a person experiencing pain. This does not mean that they should not be taken seriously or afforded respect when they tell you they are in pain. Pain is subjective and we cannot therefore make judgements about *when* someone is in pain, only *how*.
- *Confusion* can occur for a number of reasons and not all are so obvious that we can quickly assume the cause. Toxicity of any substance can cause confusion, including alcohol and illegal substances, but this must never be assumed without further

investigation. Other physical conditions that may cause confusion include dehydration, diabetes, lack of oxygen, infection, delirium, dementia, trauma to the head and psychological trauma such as post-traumatic stress disorder (PTSD).

- *Sensory impairment* can cause a general lack of understanding if information is communicated inappropriately. Someone who is deaf or blind may need information to be adapted or attending and listening skills may need to be developed in the practitioner. Using telephones and even electronic communication can sometimes help overcome this problem, while some people may prefer information that they can visualize either in the form of a film, picture or book. Some areas of practice are using mobile phone text messaging as a way of keeping in touch with clients but this may be unsuitable for the assessment stage.

- *Specific learning disabilities* such as dyslexia may cause numerical, visual and reading difficulties when communicating information, especially if it requires the person to work out a mathematical problem and record any observations. It can sometimes be taken for granted that we all have the same basic communication skills and these are easily masked or compensated for by adults who have learned to cope with deficiencies over many years.

- *Severe learning disabilities* and/or acquired brain injury can make communication difficult but should not be a reason for not communicating the care plan. The Mental Capacity Act 2005 suggests that carers should and can be consulted if this is the case, rather than not addressing the individual's needs at all. The carer however has no right to make decisions on behalf of the client unless there is a lasting power of attorney in place.

- *Anxiety and fear* can also affect how people take in information as their senses will be alert to any dangers that are present and possibly not to the information you are trying to share with them. It may be necessary to make sure you meet with the person in a safe environment for you both so that anxiety and fear do not get in the way of the assessment process. If there is any reason to suspect that this may cause problems it is important to share your concerns with a manager who has a duty to keep everyone safe under health and safety law.

- *Cultural and individual diversity* is a much neglected area in health and social care which is more often due to ignorance than contempt. We all have a responsibility to hear the person's story and what influences their beliefs. Saying 'don't be silly' is neglectful practice if we choose to ignore a person's preferences and we should at all times be responsive to individual needs. These may include basic everyday rituals and practices in relation to space, prayer, dress, diet, relationships and activities.

Abusive practice and/or neglect can occur when any of the above are not taken into consideration and not addressed within the individual's care plan. The DoH (2000b: 9) has issued guidance concerning what constitutes abuse which is helpful because some types of abuse are not as obvious as others.

- *Physical abuse* includes kicking, biting, scratching, punching, hitting, misuse of medication, restraint or inappropriate sanctions.

- *Sexual abuse* includes any acts of rape or sexual assault.
- *Psychological abuse* includes emotional abuse such as threats of harm or abandonment, humiliation, blaming, harassment, coercion, intimidation or withdrawal from services or supportive networks.
- *Financial abuse* includes theft, fraud, exploitation, pressure in connection with wills, property inheritance or financial transactions, misuse of property, possessions or benefits.
- *Neglect* includes acts of omission, failure to provide access to services and withholding medication or other treatment, such as food and heating.
- *Discriminatory abuse* includes racism, sexism, discrimination against disability, harassment or slurs connected with same.

While it is not suggested that abuse in practice is a frequent occurrence, sometimes in the busy everyday lives of practitioners it is difficult to identify when abuse may have occurred until a complaint is made or, worse, a tragedy happens. Good quality care is dependent on practitioners being able to identify some of these risks in advance so that they can be addressed and prevented quickly and efficiently.

The above outline of abusive practice is not meant to leave you with a negative view of health and social care provision. It is simply there to alert you to the dangers of ignoring abusive practice which can in some cases lead to tragic consequences. Not all individuals are aware of what abusive practice looks like (especially if they have previously been in abusive relationships) and so it is the responsibility of the practitioner to recognize it and alert people whenever they think it may be evident.

## Documentation skills: recording the information

The information you have gathered will need to be recorded as soon as possible. Ideally it should be while the person is talking but some practitioners find this difficult to do and listen/observe at the same time. The golden rule for documenting any information is therefore *as soon as possible*. The longer you leave it the harder it will be to remember, so is it is good practice to get into the habit early. Dziegielewski (2004) suggests that documenting a record of the assessment process also provides evidence for the quality of care provided. Other reasons for documenting the assessment include:

- to provide a record that the assessment has been completed, by whom and when;
- to provide a baseline for future reviews;
- to provide the information for writing up the health and social care plan;
- to provide a benchmark for the measurement of health and social care outcomes.

Assessment is an important first step in any care planning process so it is important to be clear about what you are doing, why and when it was done. This information may need to be referred to at a later date and will most certainly be required for the other stages of the care planning process. However, assessment never really ends but continues throughout the care planning process. The main issues to address at this stage are listening to and involving the client in identifying needs that you can begin to work on in the rest of the process.

## Activity 2.4

Joan has been admitted to hospital after she collapsed at home. She is known to have a serious problem with how much alcohol she consumes. You have been asked to help Joan with her lunch as a balanced diet is important for someone who uses too much alcohol. You notice a large bruise around her wrist and when you ask her about it she cannot remember how she got it. She refuses to eat much of her lunch and after trying hard to coax her you take her plate away. What should you do next?

a) Discuss with your colleagues your concerns about Joan's bruise and her lack of appetite
b) Discuss your concerns with your manager
c) Make a quick mental note to do the above and move on to helping the next patient
d) Make a quick written note in Joan's documentation about how much she has eaten and the size, shape and colour of the bruise.

The best answer is (d) because although you should discuss your concerns with your colleagues and manager they may forget what you have said or not ask enough information to make a written record later. It is best to record all information as soon as you can and due to time constraints as quickly as you can. You should therefore try and record only information that is factual and measurable wherever possible. Your opinion of how and why Joan did not eat much food or acquired the bruise is not important at this stage. Although this was an informal assessment, further formal assessment will be required to confirm the cause. However, as you have recorded the initial or 'baseline' measurement, future assessments will be able to measure any improvement or decline in Joan's health.

## Chapter summary

➡ Assessment is important to identify a person's needs and this should be as broad and holistic as possible.
➡ Informal assessment is ongoing, provides support and supplies supplementary information and modification over time.
➡ There may be barriers that will influence your assessment and these should be identified as soon as possible.
➡ Good communication skills are critical for developing a trusting relationship and eliciting the required information.
➡ Documentation completes the assessment process and ensures information is safely conveyed to other practitioners.

## Self-assessment questions

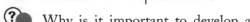 Why is it important to develop a therapeutic relationship?

Ⓠ What are the basic skills of communication?

Ⓠ Why is it important to record the care planning process?

Ⓠ What might alienate a person from the professional staff?

# 3 Planning care with the individual in need

---

**This chapter will help you to:**

➡ Explore the planning stage of the process.
➡ Discuss the role of the multidisciplinary team.
➡ Identify barriers to effective planning of care.
➡ Outline the need for evidence-based practice.
➡ Demonstrate how to plan goals.

## Introduction

> *I believe each of us working in the field of human relationships has a similar problem in knowing how to use such research knowledge. We cannot slavishly follow such findings in a mechanical way or we destroy the personal qualities which these very studies show to be valuable. It seems to me that we have to use these studies, testing them against our own experience and forming new and further hypotheses to use and test in our own further personal relationships.*

> (Rogers 1967: 50)

In Chapter 2 we identified that there are many influences on the care planning process which you should be aware of, including good communication skills, barriers to effective assessment, environmental issues and the therapeutic relationship. It is important to have this awareness so that when you come to carry out a care plan that has been written by another practitioner, you will be able to understand why you are doing a certain activity with a person in a certain way. You may not be at a stage in your development that allows you to write care plans alone, but with supervision and support you may be asked to provide information that will inform a care plan or even be offered the opportunity to write one yourself. As you were involved in the assessment of the person needing help you will also need to know how that information is transformed into achievable steps to aid their recovery and independence. This activity will also be influenced by your colleagues, your manager, the person you are carrying out the activity with, their family and quite possibly their wider social network. In Chapter 1 it was identified how philosophy models and frameworks around the whole health and social care planning process can be very influential on a successful outcome. When identifying the goals that the person needs to achieve you will need to consider these influences in detail in order for the care plan to be successful. This chapter will explore some of those influences in more detail and by the end you will be able to contribute to the areas of your practice outlined in the learning outcomes above.

## Developing the empowerment model of care planning

In Chapter 1 an empowerment model of care planning was introduced that focused on three main areas of practice using a holistic approach. This model included the core activities which should be evident throughout the care planning process:

➡ person-centred care;
➡ identifying strengths and diversity;
➡ team working.

The model was attached to the APIE framework in Chapter 2 to help us put into practice our skills and knowledge in planning care for an individual with identified health and social care needs. Figure 3.1 shows how this will look by the time we get to the planning stage.

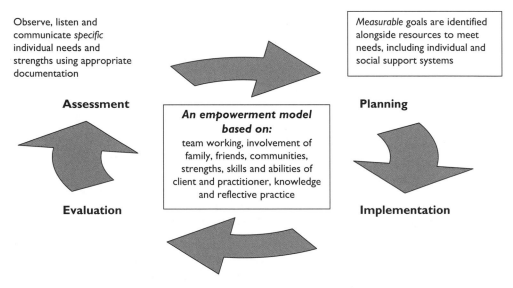

**Figure 3.1** The planning stage of the care planning process

## What is planning?

The overall aspects of planning care involve a variety of resources including time, staff, equipment, skills and knowledge, and it is your manager's responsibility to ensure that you have enough resources to carry out your work effectively and efficiently. However, your manager will not be able to provide resources until they have been requested and you or your colleagues have given good reasons or evidence for their requirement. Immediately following the person's assessment of need, therefore, it must be considered when planning their care who or what will need to be involved and why. The team will then need to prioritize resources based on the risks of dependence, safety and resource allocation which are described in more detail below. Finally, you will also need to make sure that the person for whom the care is being planned is fully involved in the whole process (or their carer if they are unable to participate), to ensure that the care plan remains focused on the client's needs in helping them recover. To begin planning care, then, we need to know what resources are available to us.

## The multidisciplinary team

Often, when we talk about planning care we talk about the 'individual care plan'. This is an outline of what the person who needs health and social care can expect to receive to help them regain their independence and/or begin recovery. However, in reality there are many other people involved who have a stake in whether the care plan is carried out correctly and in a timely way. These stakeholders are also known as the 'multidisciplinary team' and might include some or all of those identified in Figure 3.2.

### The role of the multidisciplinary team within the care plan

Figure 3.2 shows some of the main people who may be involved in the multidisciplinary team. There are other services that may also be involved but they tend to work outside health and social care settings; however, this does not detract from the fact that they may need to be involved. They include housing, education, criminal justice, welfare, benefits and probation services. Some practitioners may identify working with these satellite services as 'inter-agency' working rather than 'multidisciplinary' working and the two terms are often used interchangeably.

---

**Practice point: identifying the multidisciplinary team**

Different teams involve different people so the multidisciplinary team will not be the same in every area of practice. However, it might be worthwhile in your own area of work to think about how many people are involved in the multidisciplinary team. They may be people you see infrequently but nevertheless play an important role in care planning. Administration staff who may not be directly involved in care planning are a very important part of this process and are often the people who ensure that it all runs smoothly.

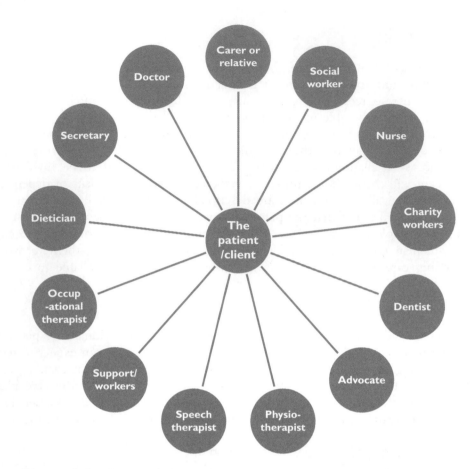

**Figure 3.2** Some of the main members of a multidisciplinary team

Multidisciplinary team members all have a responsibility to ensure that their part of the care plan is carried out. It is important therefore that the assessment and planning stages have been carried out correctly so that there is enough information for the team to work with. Often it is a lack of information and/or the communication of that information among the team that is at fault when things go wrong.

In this chapter we look closely at how the team will work together to carry out the care plan. Allison (2005) suggests that there are values and attitudes within the *partnership working* relationship that are similar to the *therapeutic relationship* that we develop with the person in need of our help. These components include:

- *Honesty* – this not only means being honest with the client or patient and each other member of the team but also honesty in providing resources and information. A client does not have to be provided with all the information about everything, as this would be too overwhelming, but they do need information that will help them make informed decisions about their health and social care needs. This may not be so easy if we find communication difficult with the client or another member of the team.

- *Candour* – this includes an awareness of confidentiality issues in that information about the patient should not be shared with everyone. However, we are required to share information if it is in the patient's best interests. This necessitates an element of trust among the team that information will only be shared for this reason but must be shared in order to carry out the care plan. Sometimes professional rivalry can get in the way of this aspect.
- *Competence* – we must all declare to our supervisors or managers if we do not feel competent to carry out a particular aspect of the care plan. This is not demonstrating a weakness but strength in one's ability to recognize one's own limits. Most professionals are bound by their professional codes of conduct to do this. It also includes making an effort to keep up to date with new interventions and resources as part of your CPD.
- *Diligence* – this is one area where practitioners and professionals must all work together to monitor for a change in circumstances and to recognize when to inform the rest of the team. While diligence is closely linked to competence it is different in that it is also linked to the assessment of a person's condition and a recognition that their needs may be decreasing or, more importantly, increasing over time.
- *Loyalty* – loyalty to the person in need of our help is a fundamental part of our work as is loyalty to our employers, managers and the rest of the team. Sometimes, however, the different expectations from the different relationships that we have in health and social care practice can lead to conflict. This will be difficult to manage but based upon the above components should be handled with help and supervision from the rest of the team. It is here that making team decisions becomes so important as these issues can be discussed together in a safe environment.
- *Fairness* – loyalty to your practice requires that you work in a fair and competent way. This may not necessarily involve the distribution of resources in a fair way but is more about the way we treat each individual person. We must not discriminate against another person, whether they are a member of our own team or a person who needs our help. We must always consider that everybody has a right to the services that we provide, whether we personally judge them to be deserving of them or not.
- *Discretion* – while we must always be aware of confidentiality it was suggested above that there will be times when we have to share information. Discretion is needed when deciding how much information needs to be shared and this should only be about areas that are relevant to the care plan. Providing information to other people about the client's standard of living or lifestyle choices is not always appropriate or necessary.

In your own area of practice there may be other people involved in planning health and social care who can affect the way a care plan is carried out. It is important therefore to think carefully about how you and the person in need of care will negotiate with other people what they can do to help the patient recover their independence and what will be realistically achievable for them. No matter how well written a care plan is, it is only as good as what it can achieve and should never knowingly be written in a way that includes goals that are unachievable. This will only set all those people involved up to fail and a new care plan will need to be written, wasting valuable time and resources. How to involve other people in the care plan will be discussed in more detail in the next chapter on implementation but you will need to consider very early on some of the practical barriers to effective care planning.

---

**Activity 3.1**

John is a middle-aged man who is trying to stop smoking; he is overweight and has developed breathing problems. He relies on his wife to do many of his daily activities for him and has been unable to work for some time. You are asked by your mentor to organize a meeting at which all the people involved in his care can discuss with Jon and his wife how they might be able to help him regain some independence. Think about the barriers to partnership working that might prevent the meeting taking place or key people attending. For example, how might you overcome the following potential barriers?

➡ A place to meet being available
➡ The time of the meeting being suitable for everyone
➡ Transport being available to attend the meeting
➡ Inviting stakeholders to attend
➡ Relevant information being available such as test and assessment results

---

Any one of the barriers to partnership working identified in Activity 3.1 could prevent a care planning meeting taking place which could then limit the amount of help John will receive. Therefore, whenever we are in a position to consult with other members of the team, however diverse or minimal, it is important that we make every effort to do so.

## Prioritizing health and social care needs

You may find setting up meetings a difficult task to manage and may need to act more quickly to provide some help in the first instance. Prioritizing care is therefore a way of managing the *risks* that are presented if nothing is done about care provision or some of the partnership working barriers identified above are getting in the way of effective care planning. For example, this is often a problem when discharge planning or changes to the initial health and/or social care plan are taking place. This is because it can be very difficult getting a group of professionals together at the same time, and careful planning will be required to work out how to do this and when will be the most suitable time for professionals, carers and clients to meet. This will also be based on the initial assessment and you may need to refer back to the outline of assessment areas that is provided in that document. Prioritizing health and social care will also need to be carried out for the group of people that you are working with as well as each individual within that group, and this may change the focus of your priorities. The following areas will help you identify and manage the needs identified in the assessment.

## Prioritizing and managing needs

- *Level of need* – the individual or group of people you are helping will all have various levels of dependence and needs that will range from needing minimal help in some areas to needing total care in all areas of their day-to-day life. You will need to prioritize care according to these needs and ensure that the more dependent people are fully supported. The safety of the person you are helping is often a way of prioritizing dependency needs – for example, a person who has mobility problems or needs help with physical or psychological difficulties may not be able to take full care of themselves. Personal supervision (Ghaye 2000; Hawkins and Shohet 2006) with a more experienced practitioner or your manager will help you with prioritization issues.
- *Risk* – there are many risks that people take with their own health and social care needs that are largely their own responsibility (e.g. smoking, overeating, lack of exercise, drinking too much alcohol etc.). Your code of conduct will suggest that providing you have offered the opportunity for information and/or support in managing these risks, the people who need help have the final decision on what type of help they will accept. This may be difficult for many of us to understand because we all have our own standards of living that may not be the same as the person we are helping. The only way that we can prioritize their safety is when the risk of them coming to some harm is greater than their ability to manage that risk. This is often evident in people with mental health problems but also in children, older, confused people and people who, through impairment or illness, are unable to help themselves. The Mental Capacity Act 2005 is useful in helping us manage risk and there are DoH publications that guide local policy on managing risk (DoH 2007a, 2008a)
- *Availability of resources* – after the initial assessment has been carried out you will have some idea of what the people you are working with need to recover their independence. In an ideal world all the resources that they need would be available (e.g. money, accommodation, social support, healthy food etc.). In reality of course, this is often not the case and we need to be flexible with the resources that we do have. You may need to explore with the patient what resources are available and adapt them somehow to meet their needs immediately rather than make them wait for any help at all. This may mean that resources are spread more thinly (e.g. a physiotherapist is only available once a week), or that they are targeted towards the most needy. This is often termed *rationing* of health and social care, but is required

to make sure that limited resources are made available to those most in need. Your manager will be able to help you obtain resources where they are available and direct you to other resources where they are not (e.g. another agency). This is another area for discussion in supervision that will support your practice and help you to prioritize your time, skills and resources. *Clinical and social governance* (discussed in more detail in Chapter 7) will also help you to prioritize resources.

---

## Activity 3.2

In Chapter 2 we identified that Brian had needs in the following areas:

**Psychological**
Managing diabetes, diet and sleep patterns. Poor mobility due
to pains in legs

**Spiritual**
Lacks belief in himself to manage his health and
social care needs and to be a valued member of
society

**Social**
Lack of social networks, some support
from brother but transport a problem as
now not driving, difficulty accessing
services

**Psychological**
Feels like life is difficult to manage, does
not have many activities since finishing
work, does not take very good care of
himself due to low self-esteem

How would you prioritize Brian's needs based on the areas identified above? (The care plan provided later in this chapter will help you to test your answers.) Remember to consider the following:

➡ Level of need
➡ Risk
➡ Availability of resources

---

## Client involvement

The involvement of clients and their carers is no longer an option according to government policy. There is an expectation for the client and their carer(s) to be visible in all aspects of planning, from individualized care plans to organizational recruitment and development. As practitioners we need to be thinking all the time about *how* and *if* we are involving clients and carers in planning care and in maintaining their personhood (Kitwood 1997; Tones 2001; Greenstreet 2006). As well as team working, this is one of the underpinning factors in planning effective care. The ways in which clients and their carers can be involved may be very diverse and because of their needs they may not be able to contribute in traditional ways, such as formal meetings and care planning reviews. As practitioners we need to be thinking of as many ways as possible of involving clients and their carers in planning care and in obtaining the best available evidence to support the care plan. The process may involve:

- group meetings or focus groups, which are often used to research the needs of a certain group;
- obtaining client and carer feedback on local or national policy documents;
- telephone interviewing/assessment;
- pre-meeting sessions to prioritize goals;
- patient satisfaction surveys;
- advocacy or befriending schemes;
- providing interpretation services for people from ethnic minorities;
- one-to-one or protected time in busy wards and/or practices.

It is generally agreed that working together in partnership between practitioners, clients and carers will lead to a greater understanding of the main needs of a group or individual and better communication in addressing those needs as agreed goals to be achieved in the long or short term (Carnwell and Buchanan 2005; Tummey 2005). The process of client and carer involvement is nevertheless still quite new in many areas of practice and requires a cultural shift in ways of working if it is to become successful. The following quote from a client suggests that there are still many barriers to full participation in care planning:

> *The systems and processes that devalue people with impairments are not consciously formulated and written down as policy, as in the case of the public services analogy, but are rooted in historical attitudes (as in the case of racism and sexism) and reinforced by both physical and social structures.*

(Minhas 2005: 73)

Kitwood (1997) carried out some very useful work with people who suffer from dementia which eventually led to a very successful dementia care mapping programme. He found that people who suffer from dementia are often ignored when planning their care because practitioners see the illness as a barrier to their involvement. He termed this 'malignant social psychology' (p. 46), and from further observations identified the following behaviours of exclusion among groups of staff. These behaviours could apply to all people that practitioners believe are unable to participate in their own care planning.

- *Deceptive* – by trying to distract or force a person into doing something without offering choices.
- *Disempowering* – taking control away from people or preventing them from achieving tasks alone.
- *Patronizing* – treating people as being like children or inadequate in making their own decisions.
- *Threatening* – suggesting that unpleasant consequence will result if the person does not comply.
- *Categorizing* – treating people as a group with an illness or disability rather than as individuals.
- *Outcasting* – treating people as if they are not liked.
- *Pressurizing* – giving information too fast and demanding a decision.
- *Unacknowledgement* – of the person's individual needs, feelings or wishes.
- *Alienation* – treating the person as if they were not human or as if they were an object.
- *Exclusion* – sending the person away or to another room, or not inviting them to a meeting.
- *Refusal* – to accept the person or give attention to their needs when requested.
- *Blaming* – the person for their behaviour instead of observing for the underlying cause.
- *Making fun* – of the person and using humour that humiliates rather than accepts them.
- *Interrupting* – the person before they have had chance to explain themselves or their needs.
- *Criticism* – by informing the person of their inadequacies rather than focusing on their strengths.

When everyday practice becomes focused on illness or disability there is a high risk that we will unknowingly ignore the needs of others or disregard them altogether. This includes the needs of staff as well as the people that we provide care for. We therefore need to be accountable for our practice at all times and able to reflect upon and justify why we have acted in a certain way when planning care. Demonstrating why we have chosen one approach over another and how this relates to the individual needs of the person will help us remain true to a person-centred approach. The evidence for the care plan therefore needs to be made available to our colleagues and to the individual and their family. This evidence will vary for each practitioner depending on their professional background (e.g. social work, nursing, occupational therapy, psychology etc.). However, it is the *quality* of the evidence that is important in that it supports our practice and ultimately the *quality* of care provided.

## Evidence-based practice

When planning care for and with an individual we need to have some knowledge of what the best available care is, otherwise they would not be coming to us for professional help. Choice of care will depend on our knowledge and skills, our experience and our professional background. Depending on the complexity of a patient's needs – i.e. the number of health and social care needs presented during the assessment phase – the practitioner may be able to plan care with the patient on their own or they may need the knowledge and skills of the multidisciplinary team. What a multidisciplinary teams consists of and how it functions were identified earlier in this chapter – the important thing to remember here is how to find the information that will ensure we are giving the best available health and social care: this is *evidence-based practice* and usually means that we have researched the area that the person needs help with and are able to provide them with at least some information and at best some help in addressing their needs. Lindsay (2007: xi) suggests that evidence-based practice 'Involves using the best evidence you have about the most effective care of individuals, using it with the person's best interests in mind, to the best of your ability and in such a way that it is clear to others that you are doing it'.

When planning care, it will therefore take you or your colleagues a little time to ensure that you have the best available evidence to hand should anyone ask why you are planning care in that particular way. Activity 3.3 will help you to do this.

---

**Activity 3.3**

Go to a journal within your professional field and find some research on a particular difficulty that someone might commonly experience (e.g. falls). When you have read the article, discuss with your tutor or supervisor the following questions:

(?) Does the research explore the needs of people similar to the person you are planning care with?

(?) Is the research recent and transferable to your area of practice?

(?) Does the research demonstrate any sort of bias towards certain practices (e.g. medication)?

(?) Does the research give a fair account of the results, including limitations?

If the research paper can answer all of the above questions to your satisfaction then it will probably be useful to you in your practice and you will be able to justify your care planning decisions based upon the best available care.

---

Hierarchy of evidence

Even when we do provide evidence for our practice we must be aware of the *hierarchy of evidence* that is available to us. This means that some evidence is thought to be better than others simply because it has been through more stringent methods of collection and analysis. While it could be (and is) argued that some methods of research are not appropriate for use with human beings, there still appears to be a 'gold standard' of evidence that is applied to all research whether it is appropriate or not. Lindsay (2007) argues that this relates to what is known as 'positivist research' or research that can reduce the information collected to reliable information that can be transferred elsewhere with the same result (e.g. wound care: most people would agree on what recent evidence there is available about the most effective healing methods). Lindsay (2007: 39) provides a hierarchy of such positivist research or evidence, as follows, beginning with the most rigorous method:

❶ *Systematic review* – research that looks at all the available research on a given topic.
❷ *Randomized controlled trial (RCT)* – research that tries to control as many factors as possible (e.g. age of participants).
❸ *Quasi-experimental study* – not as controlled as an RCT but having some controls.
❹ *Non-systematic literature review* – can be selective.
❺ *Expert opinion* – most often a consultant in the field.

With the exception of expert opinion, the above are known as *quantitative methods* in that there is usually some way of measuring or quantifying the results. Alternatively, and more frequently in the health and social care professions, *qualitative* research methods are used to elicit the experiences of people who use services in order to improve the service provided (Elliott 2005).

As practitioners we are not always expected to know how to carry out research, and many practitioners never do. We are expected, however, to have some understanding of how research informs our practice and we must learn to understand the rigour of the different approaches (M. Smith 2004). Once we have overcome our fear of research, we can use it to our advantage in supporting our claims for the resources needed to carry out the care plan. Knowledge of research also gives us confidence that we are organizing the best possible care for our clients. Useful sources for reliable research include:

- The National Institute for Health and Clinical Excellence (NICE).
- The Social Care Institute for Excellence (SCIE).
- The National Institute for Mental Health England (NIMHE).

Journals are also an invaluable source of the most up-to-date research in your field of work. You may have used one of these when completing Activity 3.3. However, don't restrict yourself solely to journals in your field: very often other related fields produce papers that contain elements of crossover between disciplines.

## The skills of planning care

In the planning stage we need to translate identified needs into goals or outcomes that can be measured during the implementation and evaluation stages. It is important to acknowledge at this stage that plans must only be made that are specific, measurable, achievable, realistic and timely (SMART) (NTA 2006). The acronym SMART is used to help us remember this when planning care or any sort of intervention:

- *Specific* – in what form, when and how will the care be provided?
- *Measurable* – how will the care be measured and what tools will be used to achieve this (e.g. a score to be achieved on an assessment tool)?
- *Achievable* – are resources/staff in place to implement the care plan and will it be put into effect as soon as possible?
- *Realistic* – is the plan realistic? Some goals may require small steps to be achieved before the main aim is accomplished (e.g. going out alone may require other resources to be available such as walking aids and the knowledge and confidence to use them).
- *Timely* – is there a realistic time frame in place to ensure that there has been every opportunity for change to have taken place?

If we do not consider a SMART approach to planning health and social care then no matter how wonderful the care plan may look it is highly unlikely to be successful. When planning care it is always necessary to take some time to consider with the client what expectations can be realistically achieved. This part of the care plan is rather like a contract between the client and the practitioner and will involve some elements of negotiation and compromise.

Writing out this section of the care plan involves identifying the realistic goals or outcomes that both you and your client agree on. It is important to remember before you even start to write down these goals or outcomes that if they are not identified in agreement with the client and the team, the whole care plan may become unachievable. This is not the sign of good care planning skills and immediately draws attention to a lack of careful thought concerning the care plan. There is much criticism of care planning being a 'paper exercise' that takes the practitioner away from their work with people. However, if carried out correctly, care planning will help you keep focused on what you both need to be doing in order to restore independence and recovery. Creating dependence on a service as a result of poor care planning not only contributes to a heavier cost to the health and social care budget but can also lead to 'burnout' among staff and patients when they fail to achieve unrealistic goals. It is always better to develop small 'step-wise' goals than goals that could take a lifetime to achieve. The Open University (1997) suggests that behavioural goals are more measurable and should be considered when planning care. Behavioural goal-setting involves:

- identifying the person(s) who will achieve the goal;
- identifying the behaviour that will be demonstrated;
- identifying the conditions for the behaviour to occur;
- identifying measures for evaluating the behaviour;
- identifying how often or by when the behaviour is to be achieved.

## Writing goals into the care plan

We have now agreed with Brian that he needs support in certain key areas (see Activity 3.2 for a quick reminder). When we come to write these needs in his care plan we must remember to prioritize them in order of importance. This order will be influenced by the risk assessment. We will then need to decide what can realistically be achieved in the short term and in the long term.

### Short- and long-term goals

Some people who have complex care needs may identify goals that they want to achieve immediately and goals that they would like to achieve in the future. These are short- and long-term goals. The most obvious clue as to which is which is the time over which the person expects to achieve the goal, but some are so long term (and ambitious) that they may take years to achieve. This is not helpful if we are to instil hope that the person can recover and gain some independence. It is therefore useful to insert some short-term easy-to-achieve goals into any care plan so that people can see that a change has taken place and take heart for the future.

The care plan is a legal document and acts as a communication tool between all those involved in the person's care. It therefore needs to be specific enough to convey the right message and must be measurable so that it can be properly evaluated. The Open University (1997: 50) suggests that if goals are not stated clearly and written SMART-ly then the result will be 'fuzzy goals' that may be open to interpretation by other people. Here are some examples:

- 'reduce breathlessness';
- 'relieve pain';
- 'provide reassurance'.

For Brian, fuzzy goals might be:

- 'alleviate pain';
- 'stabilize diabetes';
- 'provide information on diabetes';
- 'improve sleep pattern'.

You can see that these goals would be difficult to measure and therefore do not represent a good quality care plan. There are probably many more such fuzzy goals out there but it is our task to eliminate them as much as possible and to write goal statements with the client and/or the multidisciplinary team that are SMART. For Brian we have identified that we can:

- measure when his diabetes has stabilized by recording regular blood sugar levels;
- record pain levels as identified by Brian and report them to the physiotherapist/ consultant and other relevant professionals;

- identify, support and discuss information on managing Brian's diabetes;
- assess and monitor Brian's sleep patterns in hours and quality;
- increase local social networks and community support networks for Brian.

All of the above short-term goals are recordable and measurable to demonstrate progress made during the care planning process. They are written into the care plan as shown below.

## Care plan using the **SMART** formula

| Patient name Brian Jones | | Date of birth 01/01/1955 | |
| --- | --- | --- | --- |
| **Needs** (*specific: in person's own words where possible*) | **Goals** (*measurable and achievable: including any assessment tool measurements*) | **Interventions** (*realistic*) | **Evaluation** (*timely*) |
| *1. Help with managing diabetes* | **Short-term goal** *To stabilize diabetes with the help of the practice nurse, dietician and GP*  **Long-term goal** *For Brian to maintain a healthy diet that reduces fluctuations in blood sugar levels and attend regular appointments with services* | | |
| *2. Help with mobility* | **Short-term goal** *GP and physiotherapist to assess and alleviate reported pain levels, currently 6 out of 10*  **Long-term goal** *For Brian to feel less pain on moving and to be able to attend meetings and socialize more frequently* | | |

| | | | |
|---|---|---|---|
| 3. Low mood | **Short-term goal** <br> Care coordinator to provide and discuss information on how to manage the condition <br><br> **Long-term goal** <br> For Brian to be more in control of his life and his future | | |
| 4. Sleep excess | **Short-term goal** <br> Care coordinator to assess and monitor sleep pattern <br><br> **Long-term goal** <br> For Brian to sleep less and have more time in the day to take care of himself | | |
| 5. Lacks social support | **Short-term goal** <br> Social worker to increase access to social networks <br><br> **Long-term goal** <br> For Brian to have a wider support network to help him self-care by increasing contacts with other organizations/people | | |
| *Signatures* | Care coordinator <br><br> A.N. Other, Registered Nurse | Client <br><br> Brian Jones | Date <br><br> 01/02/10 |

## Communicating the care plan

Recording everything that you have done in the daily record sheet is required for reviewing and evaluating Brian's care plan but also provides information for other people who will be implementing part of, or the entire, care plan. These may be people you are passing Brian's care over to on a day-to-day basis, the multidisciplinary team or people who are commissioning his care. The importance of communicating the care plan cannot be overstated. In the next chapter we will explore in more detail how this can be achieved.

## Chapter summary

➡ Following assessment there must be a written plan of care that includes as many stakeholders or members of the multidisciplinary team as required.

➡ The care coordinator in liaison with the team and the person being assessed will devise the areas of priority for the care plan using the best available evidence.

➡ Prioritization is important in identifying risk, dependency and resources.

➡ Goals should be written in a way that clearly outlines what needs to happen and when.

➡ The care plan must be communicated and negotiated with all those involved including the client and their carers where necessary.

## Self-assessment questions

What is the role of the multidisciplinary team in care planning?

How can we prioritize health and social care needs effectively?

How can we make sure clients are involved in their care plan?

What barriers might there be to effective care planning?

# 4 Implementing the planned care

This chapter will help you to:

→ Identify the role of the practitioner in implementing the care plan.
→ Understand the importance of reflective practice.
→ Understand the knowledge and skills needed to implement a care plan.
→ Identify the importance of record-keeping.

## Introduction

> *The role of the health professional is not so much to ferret out the innermost secrets (which can easily lend itself to a dangerous kind of voyeurism) as it is to assist the chronically ill and those around them to come to terms with – that is accept, master or change – those personal significances that can be shown to be operating in their lives and in their care. I take this to constitute the essence of what is now called empowering patients.*

(Kleinman 1988: 43)

The implementation stage (see Figure 4.1) is the point where all the elements of the care plan worked out to date are put into effect. As with all the previous stages, the eventual outcome will depend on the skill and commitment of the individual care team members, and on the resources with which they are provided.

There are some differences between implementing care for patients in a residential setting and those living in the community, but there are equally some basic principles that apply to both settings, and these are identified below. The first thing to remember at this point is that implementing care does not just 'happen'. Planning and monitoring are necessary and are the responsibility of the team leader, care coordinator, manager or ward sister, as appropriate, with the support of the multidisciplinary team. For the purpose of this chapter we will call this person the *care coordinator*. Their responsibility is to make sure the care plan is carried out when needed and not just when it is convenient for the individual practitioner or team. This can cause some conflict when each member of the team is trying to ensure that each person they are planning care for receives the best quality care available. It is necessary therefore for the care coordinator to develop skills, knowledge and attitudes that will help them carry out their role.

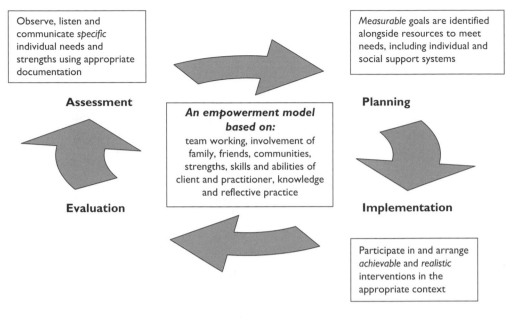

**Figure 4.1** Implementation stage

At the implementation stage all your knowledge and skills are brought together. In particular, your ability to make and maintain relationships with a variety of people will be put to the test. However, as a newly-developing practitioner you will not be expected to know everything about everything, but you will be expected to know where to find out information and how to use it. For example, you will need to draw upon the main policies and guidelines for each individual patient/client and in particular how each member of the team applies them. Only when the team is working together in a harmonized way will the care plan be delivered effectively. Allison (2005) believes that the attributes of honesty, candour, competence, diligence, loyalty, fairness and discretion are important in multidisciplinary team working (see Chapter 3).

---

**Activity 4.1**

Find out what policies are in place where you work with regard to care planning for clients. If there are none, discuss this with your mentor or manager. It is always important to become familiar with local policies on care delivery, both for your own professional benefit and that of your patients.

## The skills of the care coordinator

A care coordinator needs to develop the following skills to be successful in their role.

### Decision-making

The care coordinator will need to be able to make decisions about whether the care being provided is adequate and whether on a day-to-day basis anything needs to change. For example, there may be a problem with obtaining a particular medicine or dressing. As it is impossible to call the whole team together on such a frequent basis it is the care coordinator who makes these decisions, preferably in consultation with the client. If the client is too ill to be actively involved, the care coordinator should be in a position to assess who else it would be suitable to consult (e.g. carers).

### Empathy and reflective practice

Developing an empathic approach towards helping people make decisions involves good listening and questioning skills as well as good reflective skills. An empathic care coordinator will be constantly reflecting on the care plan with the client and their own supervisor(s) to ensure everyone has a shared understanding of what is happening. Jaspers (2003: 1) suggests that reflective practice

> is different from acquiring skills by watching others and mimicking what they do because it involves constantly thinking about and actively making decisions. Hence reflective practice bridges the gap between pure theory and directed practice by providing a strategy that helps to develop understanding and learning.

### The role of supervision

When this type of reflective practice is carried out with another person or persons it is sometimes known as 'management', 'clinical' or 'peer' supervision. Supervision sessions are usually held at least once a month and the outcome documented in the care plan. The supervision process is often a requirement of professionals as part of their code of conduct. Supervision can also act as a protection measure against the everyday turbulence of practice. Hawkins and Shohet (2006: 3) identify that:

> We have often seen very competent workers reduced to severe doubt about themselves and their abilities to function in their work through absorbing disturbance from their clients. The supervisor's role is not just to reassure the worker but to allow the emotional disturbance to be felt within the safer setting of a supervisory relationship where it can be survived, reflected upon and learnt from.

Good interpersonal skills will therefore help you to voice your concerns if you feel that the care plan is not working and make changes to improve the likelihood that it will. A model of reflection is provided further on in this chapter and supervision is discussed in more detail in the next chapter.

## Organizational skills

Managing time is a major constraint when planning how best to deliver high standards of care. Some decisions about the organization of the day are beyond our control, such as the need for rest, meals, therapeutic activities, outpatient appointments etc. These aspects of a day often appear to interfere with person-centred care but still need to be carried out to maintain the smooth running of the care plan. However, without some kind of organized activity the health and social care team would not be able to function.

---

### Activity 4.2

Take some time to reflect on your daily routine. How much of it is organized by someone else and how much are you responsible for? Consider your whole working day and make a list in the boxes below. Try to be completely honest with yourself.

| Activities that I organize | Activities that others organize |
| --- | --- |
|  |  |

---

By identifying what is fixed and cannot be moved and what can be changed we can more effectively plan care. For example, if a client needs exercise every day for health reasons then that should be prioritized over another client who needs exercise for social reasons. Obviously if the two people agree to have their exercise together then this would make the best use of resources. Unfortunately, in reality some care plans are not implemented because either there is a lack of resources or the plan has been written in such a way that it is totally unrealistic to achieve.

When working in a community setting it is often overlooked that there needs to be careful consideration given to travelling time. Can contact be made with the care coordinator in rural areas or is it better to make home visits in pairs? The latter is very time-consuming but must be considered as part of the risk assessment. The health and safety of all those involved in working with people in the community must be taken seriously and in particular lone working policies should be available. The Health and Safety Executive (HSE) website (www.hse.gov.uk) provides plenty of information on what to look out for in the community and in the working environment which must be taken into account when allocating time. Health and safety in the workplace is everybody's responsibility and taking shortcuts should not be an option.

## Managing the environment

Some environmental barriers to effective care planning were identified in Chapter 2. However, there are other aspects of the environment that are of particular importance when implementing a care plan. These include cleanliness, noise, distractions, heating, lighting, transport issues, communication barriers and space for rest and relaxation.

It is very important when implementing the care plan that you become aware of the environment in which you are working. You may want to talk to your supervisor about this, especially if you have identified areas for improvement. Even areas of the environment over which you have no control need to be identified in order to construct the care plan to take account of this.

---

**Activity 4.3**

Take a look around your working environment. Are there any issues that affect your ability to do your job properly? Make a list to take to your next supervision meeting.

---

*Essence of Care* (DoH 2003c: 6) highlights the following environmental 'benchmarks' to consider with carers and clients:

- *access to care* – people can access the care environment safely and easily;
- *culture: 'how it feels'* – people feel comfortable, safe, reassured, confident and welcome;
- *well maintained* – people experience care in a tidy and well-maintained area;
- *clean* – people experience care in a consistently clean environment;
- *infection control* – people feel confident that infection control precautions are in place;
- *personal* – patients' personal environment is managed to meet their individual needs;
- *linen and furnishings* – patients' care is supported by effective use of linen and furnishings.

These benchmarks are used for auditing the care environment, so it is important you become familiar with them as part of your everyday practice. If you have concerns about any of the above you should record and report them.

# Cultural diversity

In modern society it is becoming increasingly common for local communities to experience a wide difference in culture and beliefs. Many areas of a person's life can be affected by these differences and so we must never assume that we already know how a person would like to be cared for: we could be breaching their individual human rights. A lack of recognition of cultural diversity can lead to a care plan breaking down for some very simple but extremely important reasons. Examples include:

- *Communication* – are there any language barriers that may interfere with implementing the care plan? Does the client understand what is going to happen and has anyone been contacted to aid this process (e.g. an interpreter, a relative or close friend). It is always better to choose an interpreter over a relative or friend, even though this might be time-consuming to arrange, as there is a risk that a person who is close to the client may also make assumptions about their needs. Under the Mental Capacity Act 2005 and the Mental Health Act 2007 a person is entitled to an independent advocate if they are deemed unable to consent or if they choose not to involve their family or friends.

- *Time management* – does the person have any particular personal or religious routines that they need to carry out each day? This may interfere with your plans if they have not been considered in advance and the person is unavailable when you need to carry out a particular aspect of the care plan. The care plan should specify when an activity is to be carried out, at a time that is convenient to both the health professionals and the client.

- *Managing the environment* – some people need to have some of their personal possessions around them. This is especially important if such items relate to religious practice (e.g. rosary beads). Not acknowledging such a need shows a lack of respect for the individual which could have detrimental effects on any therapeutic relationship you are trying to develop. No matter how silly a personal item might appear to you, it may have great personal or religious value to the client and every attempt to accommodate the individual's wishes should be made.

- *Personal care* – preferences in this area should have been identified at the initial assessment but we should never assume that this has been done and should always check with the client before any interventions are carried out. Without gaining proper consent each personal touch could constitute abuse and/or assault. For this reason you must always gain consent for any intervention and you should explore the person's individual preferences for cleansing, spiritual and social care, food preferences and the gender of the person who is allocated to care for them. In some sensitive areas of care this is very important for successful implementation of the care plan and you may need to involve the family in this process.

**Hot topic**

Cultural diversity is sometimes only thought about in relation to different ethnic groups. This can cause problems if you are working in an area where there are no ethnic groups or there is a strong sense of cultural identity. In either case we need to be aware that some people will not fit into a generalized approach to health and social care and their individual needs must always be taken into account. We all have individual rights protected by laws such as the Human Rights Act 2000 and the Disability Discrimination Act 2005 which you may need to become more familiar with in your own area of practice.

## Implementing the care plan

If we have involved Brian and any other agencies during the assessment and planning stages we should now have a good idea of what resources/support is available for him. The section of the documentation on implementation might look something like the example shown below. Remember we still need to keep the record factual and measurable so that other people can see what Brian needs to help him recover.

| **Patient name** Brian Jones | | **Date of birth** 01/01/1955 | |
|---|---|---|---|
| **Needs** (*specific: in person's own words where possible*) | **Goals** (*measurable and achievable: including any assessment tool measurements*) | **Interventions** (*realistic*) | **Evaluation** (*timely*) |
| 1. Help with managing diabetes | **Short-term goal** *To stabilize diabetes with the help of the practice nurse, dietician and GP* <br><br> **Long-term goal** *For Brian to maintain a healthy diet that reduces fluctuations in blood sugar levels and attend regular appointments with services* | *1. Arrange regular appointments with GP/practice nurse in local surgery for close monitoring of blood sugar levels* <br> *2. Contact local diabetic support group and help Brian make initial visit* <br> *3. Provide information for Brian and his brother on self-care and any other support available* | |

| 2. Help with mobility | **Short-term goal** GP and physiotherapist to assess and alleviate reported pain levels, currently 6 out of 10 | 1. Arrange appointment with doctor to discuss pain and treatment options 2. Help Brian to attend any outpatient appointments (e.g. pain clinic, diabetes clinic, physiotherapy, occupational therapy) 3. Arrange transport to help Brian attend appointments | |
| | **Long-term goal** For Brian to feel less pain on moving and to be able to attend meetings and socialize more frequently | | |
| 3. Low mood | **Short-term goal** Care coordinator to provide and discuss information on how to manage the condition | 1. Assess mood using specific tools 2. Obtain information on self-care and discuss with Brian 3. Help Brian to access information (e.g. via internet at local library) 4. Discuss with Brian options and risks when managing his condition 5. Discuss with Brian the benefits of keeping a mood diary | |
| | **Long-term goal** For Brian to be more in control of his life and his future | | |
| 4. Sleep excess | **Short-term goal** Care coordinator to assess and monitor sleep pattern | 1. Help Brian to identify his individual sleep patterns 2. Obtain information to help Brian improve his sleep patterns 3. Discuss with Brian the benefits of keeping a sleep diary | |
| | **Long-term goal** For Brian to sleep less and have more time in the day to take care of himself | | |

| 5. Lacks social support | **Short-term goal** Social worker to increase access to social networks | 1. Identify local support networks with Brian 2. Help Brian to choose which support networks to contact/attend | |
| | **Long-term goal** For Brian to have a wider support network to help him self-care by increasing contacts with other organizations and people | 3. Help Brian to identify transport options 4. Help Brian to obtain financial support with transport costs where available | |
| Signatures | Care Coordinator A.N. Other, Registered Nurse | Client Brian Jones | Date 01/02/10 |

## Indicators of good quality care

The following aspects of our professional development are usually within our control and can help us to maintain the best possible standards of care.

- *Competence* – in order to carry out effective interventions with clients we must be as sure as possible that we are up to date with the best available evidence (Lindsay 2007). If you fear that you may not be up to date, make sure that you seek further information or advice from other professionals who are.
- *Good team-working skills* – everyone who has ever worked in a team will know how difficult this can be. Even if your immediate colleagues are in tune with each other, the wider multidisciplinary team will most certainly not be, only coming together for major reviews or evaluations of the care plan at certain intervals. It is important therefore that you develop your interpersonal skills so that you are able to provide the most relevant facts and information required for other team members to carry out their roles. This also means informing people as soon as possible about any changes to the care plan. Unfortunately, we may have to admit that we are not always very good at this part of our role. You should remember however that it is a strength of a good reflective practitioner to admit when we may not know all the answers. Hawkins and Shohet (2006: 3) suggest that 'In times of stress it is sometimes easier to keep one's head down, to get on with it and not take time to reflect. Organizations, teams and individuals can collude with this attitude for a variety of reasons including external pressures and internal fears of exposing individual inadequacies'.

Some dos and don'ts of implementing a care plan

- Do record every action in the person's notes.
- Do talk over *any* concerns with your colleagues no matter how small.
- Do make every effort to inform the team of what you are doing.
- Do consider any health and safety matters for every activity.
- Do try to reflect upon what you are doing during practice and in supervision.
- Don't be afraid to admit that you don't know everything – this is a strength not a weakness.
- Don't forget to reflect upon your practice as often as possible and make it a good practice habit.
- Don't break confidentiality if at all possible.
- Don't take any action without ensuring that you have consent.
- Don't cancel your supervision sessions if you are overworked – they are even more important at this time.

## Record-keeping

As outlined in previous chapters it is vital that we record every observation and action taken in relation to our day-to-day work with patients. These records can then be discussed when evaluating care and in supervision with your manager/mentor. It is a legal responsibility of all registered professionals to do this, but certain aspects of record-keeping may be delegated to unregistered practitioners, especially when it is the unregistered practitioner who has made contact with the patient or client: the record should then be in their own words.

Memory is not very reliable so it is important to document your findings as soon as possible after every intervention. However, it is a myth that good record-keeping means lots of words on a page. In fact, the reverse is true: the skill is to be *factual* and *frugal* with what you write.

Good record-keeping during the implementation stage is of the utmost importance. Many patient records have excellent assessment and care planning documentation but this is not always used in the most efficient way. This section will outline the most important points to remember about your record-keeping skills which you can in turn use as a self-evaluation tool. Most professional and organizational guidelines make reference to record-keeping as an *individual* responsibility, so it is important to remember that we cannot blame anyone or anything else when it has not been done, or not been done well. The code of ethics for occupational therapists (College for Occupational Therapists 2005: 10) clearly states that:

> *Occupational therapists shall accurately record all information related to their involvement with the client, as an occupational therapy record, part of a multidisciplinary record or as a client held record. This responsibility shall extend to other occupational therapy personnel in accordance with local guidelines.*

The NMC (2007) also provides detailed guidance for professionals on record-keeping.

daily record sheet provides an example of what might be recorded
lementation of Brian's care plan. Try casting an analytical eye over
e will expand on this further in this and the next few chapters.

**Daily record sheet – to be completed by care coordinator or by designated person and countersigned by care coordinator**

| Date | Record to be made at least once daily or on every contact | Signature and designation |
|---|---|---|
| 01/01/10 16.00 hours | *4. I visited Brian today at 3 p.m.*<br><br>*1. Brian has also visited his practice nurse for blood sugar monitoring today at 10 a.m.*<br><br>*3. Brian appeared more cheerful in mood stating that he had been out to watch some football with his brother. We assessed his mood using the assessment tool and he scored 15, indicating mild depression.*<br><br>*2. Brian has an appointment for 30 January at 2 p.m. to see the medical consultant (Mr Goodwin) about the pain in his legs.*<br><br>*5. I took Brian some information on self-care and discussed with him what his options might be. We also talked about what social support networks were available in the local community centre. Brian suggested that he attend the art class which is something he has always wanted to try but never had the time.* | *A.N. Other, RN* |
| | | |
| | | |

**Practice point: record-keeping skills**

Before moving on to the next part of this chapter, have a look at the record-keeping skills of your mentor or colleagues. Are their records precise, measurable and short, and do they give you enough (or too much) information?

You should have access to record-keeping polices in your area of work and it is important to become familiar with them as soon as possible. Briefly, the main points to remember are:

- record the date and time of the intervention as well as the date and time of the entry into the patient's notes – it is important to note if these differ because something could have happened in between;
- clearly sign the notes with your name and designation (job title) and obtain countersignatures if you are not the registered practitioner responsible for the care plan;
- keep to the facts: do not enter personal feelings as these are not objective (measurable);
- note any observations that are measurable (e.g. drank one mug of tea);
- note the name of anyone you have discussed the patient with (including during supervision), plus the date and time;
- note the problem or need you were addressing during your intervention (usually a number is sufficient but you will need to check if needs/problems have been numbered in the care plan);
- note any concerns that you may have about consent and capacity to consent (e.g. 'Mr X appeared confused so I informed him of the procedure again before commencement and obtained verbal consent to proceed');
- if some information or activity is not recorded it can be considered that it has not been done. This may constitute neglect at any later inquiry and now carries a prison sentence of up to five years under the Mental Capacity Act 2005.

## Reflective practice as a monitoring tool

It is important at this stage in the care plan to reflect on the progress both you and the client have made (in fact you have been reflecting on practice in every activity you have attempted so far). This is necessary because you will need to become alert to any new issues that arise and which might present a risk to Brian's care plan being carried out effectively. You need to talk with Brian in order to monitor progress and to ensure that he remains involved in the care planning process. Ensuring that his voice is heard throughout the process is part of our advocacy role but it is also an action that we can demonstrate and therefore measure. A prominent writer on reflection, Donald Schön (1983), identifies that it is difficult sometimes for practitioners to talk or become more conscious about their practice. The implementation stage is therefore difficult to measure but it is not impossible. By encouraging Brian to tell the story of his experience of the care planning process we are also ensuring that he is able to maintain access to services and support systems. This 'reflective conversation' is another skill that practitioners must develop to ensure good quality care is provided at all times (Ghaye 2000).

Although there is an identified evaluation stage there may need to be changes made to the care plan immediately that cannot wait until the plan is formally reviewed. In relation to Brian, his care plan may be working very well until one of these common problems occurs:

- a member of the team goes off sick;
- an appointment with another member of the team is cancelled or delayed;
- Brian's brother goes on holiday;
- transport does not arrive at the stated time;
- Brian does not receive the information he needs to manage his diabetes.

The above hitches cannot be planned for in advance; however, we can all learn to respond to changes by becoming more reflective about what we do in everyday practice and applying those principles when things change. Ghaye (2000) suggests that the information you gather when reflecting on your practice can be taken to supervision meetings with your manager or mentor and used as supporting information when the care plan is evaluated more formally (see Chapter 5 for more information on supervision). In the remainder of this chapter we will look at reflective practice in more detail in order to identify what skills are needed to become a reflective practitioner.

## The skills of reflective practice

There are many models of reflection that have originated from the field of education where it was recognized that if people thought in more depth about their practice it could lead to an improvement in the quality of their learning and the practice provided (Gibbs 1988). Often reflection is misunderstood as simply a way of describing what happened, but for reflective practice to be effective the practitioner needs to be able to identify the basic facts of what happened and *how* any problems were addressed, using evidence-based practice.

Jaspers (2003: 1) suggests that reflective practice helps us to bridge the theory–practice gap by providing evidence for why we do things in a particular way which might not be exactly as the textbooks tell us. She suggests that reflective practice 'involves consciously thinking about things and actively making decisions'. This implies that reflection includes some sort of action that involves more than just recording our practice. Jaspers goes on to highlight three elements of reflective practice:

- An *event* or something you can identify as having happened in your practice and which you can tell as a story to another person. For example, how you carried out a particular task or in Brian's case how you provided him with information about his diabetes.
- A *model* of reflection that will help you to explore your practice in greater detail and which usually breaks down your reflection into certain components. However, different models emphasize different theories, as discussed in Chapter 1.
- An *outcome* that results in a new viewpoint on practice based on an exploration of the evidence provided from the story and matching this with the theory and skills required to practise good quality care.

Reflective practice needs all three elements for it to be effective and therefore can only be carried out *in practice*. The client must be at the centre of any reflective practice concerning care planning because it is *their* story that we should be telling and not what we as professionals *think* they should be saying.

---

### Practice point: recording patients' stories

One way of ensuring that patients' stories are recorded properly is to use their own words wherever possible in the care planning documentation, especially in relation to how they feel about something or a particular intervention, as the words they use can alter or identify the meaning to the person and the practitioner. As practitioners we can also learn how effective the care plan is likely to be, even before it is implemented. For example, if Brian tells you he has difficulty getting off to sleep and therefore sleeps later into the morning, making him an appointment for 9.00 a.m. at the GP's surgery for his blood sugar monitoring is highly unlikely to be successful.

---

## Telling the patient's story as evidence-based practice

In Chapter 3 a hierarchy of evidence was discussed as a way of measuring the quality of our evidence-based practice (Lindsay 2007). However, not all evidence can be gleaned from the gold standard of the RCT and it is within the care plan that more qualitative research can be found on individualized person-centred care. Narrative research is becoming a more common method of gathering information and evidence that is meaningful to people's life stories (Elliott 2005). Just as each of the people we care for is a unique individual with their own needs, each of our experiences with people is unique to the given situation and can only be supported, but never completely directed, by evidence-based practice. A narrative account occurs when the views of the client and the practitioner are sought about an event and then brought together in a holistic way (Kleinman 1988). The power of storytelling in health and illness is perhaps an underused tool to demonstrate values and attitudes towards person-centred care. Kleinman (1988: 50) goes on to suggest that 'for the care giver what is important is to witness a life story, to validate its interpretation and to affirm its value'.

Narrative practice through reflection therefore gives more than one person's account and demonstrates that collaboration has taken place in the form of empowering practice (Lloyd 2009). Based on a theory of reflective practice such as that of Gibbs (1988) or Jaspers (2003), when using reflection, the practitioner needs to be able to identify that certain components have occurred which will also need to be documented in the person's records. The following EVENT framework is suitable for all areas of practice. The model is based on the theory of narrative research (Elliott 2005) but encompasses all the areas of practice that are required under clinical and social governance policy (SCIE 2007; DoH 2008b). These aspects have been highlighted in bold in Figure 4.2.

Becoming a reflective or narrative practitioner requires practice and time but will be a useful tool wherever you go in your personal and professional development. It is important therefore to get into the habit early in your career rather than waiting for some memorable event to happen. This quality development approach does not reduce a person or event to a set of facts or figures only, but expands on the basic information to provide a rich account of your practice from which you and your colleagues can continue to learn.

| Evaluate | Visualize | Evidence | Notify |
|---|---|---|---|
| *What happened* | *How to improve practice* | *For improvement* | *The client and team* |
| **Take** | | | |
| *All of the above to supervision with your manager or mentor* | | | |

**Figure 4.2** EVENT framework for reflective practice

- *Evaluate* what happened by gathering information from everyone involved including the client and carer, but be careful to gather only the facts – not opinions or feelings. It is important that you get as much information as possible and are careful not to add any attitudes or value judgements of your own.
- *Visualize* the main issues or points for further exploration. This requires narrowing down all the information that you have gathered to key issues that are significant to the people involved. A simple list of issues that need dealing with can then be created and be checked as they are addressed. This is also helpful in identifying any risks that may have become evident. Some of these issues may need to be developed into planning a policy later on if it becomes evident that they occur frequently.
- Provide *evidence* from individual experiences or research of interventions that may address the issues. This may involve some further research on your behalf, via journals, websites or the advice of professional colleagues.
- *Notify* all those involved of the action plan created to address the issue. This is where team working and staff management are really important because if changes have to be made quickly it is essential that the rest of the team involved in providing care are updated as soon as possible.
- *Take* the action plan to your next supervision session and document in the person's notes the main outcomes of your supervision. You may have already made the changes to the care plan by this stage unless it is something that requires authorization by your manager/mentor. In either case, good preparation through reflection will help you access resources quickly following authorization and/or make good use of your supervision time with your manager. Making a record of supervision also demonstrates that you have tried to address the issue and that you

have kept everyone informed. This may include a staff training issue that will need to be addressed or an individual action plan for your own CPD.

If we apply the EVENT framework to Brian, the result will be something similar to that shown in Figure 4.3.

| Evaluate | Visualize | Evidence | Notify |
|---|---|---|---|
| *Brian did not attend an appointment* | *Need to review transport arrangements for appointments* | *Poor mobility may be making it difficult for Brian to access services* | *Let the team know that transport/access is presenting a problem* |

<table>
<tr><td colspan="4" align="center">Take<br>Discuss in supervision the following:<br>How to help Brian gain better access to services<br>What has been discussed with Brian and how he thinks this issue can be improved</td></tr>
</table>

**Figure 4.3** An example of reflection on practice based on Brian's care plan

The link between reflective practice and supervision will be discussed in more detail in the next chapter but before you move on try the following activity using the EVENT framework.

---

**Activity 4.4**

Think of a situation you have been in when you have had to make decisions about your own actions. Use the EVENT framework to help you work through what happened and how you dealt with the situation. This may have been a conversation with another person or some action that you have taken regarding your own health care needs (e.g. giving up smoking, taking more exercise etc.).

➡ **Evaluate** what happened, remembering to keep to the facts only
➡ **Visualize** how you could change things to improve the situation
➡ **Evidence** the actions that you took: why did you do it that particular way, what knowledge informed your practice?
➡ **Notify** the appropriate people: who did you tell about your decision and why?
➡ **Take** to supervision and record how you did this: who are the people that you value as your mentors or guides and how did you record your actions? Do you keep a reflective journal or diary?

## Chapter summary

➡ The implementation stage of delivering care is the most important part of good quality health and social care provision and yet is probably the most unrecorded.

➡ Skills involved in implementing the care plan include good interpersonal skills, decision-making, reflection and team-working skills.

➡ Time management is essential when implementing a care plan efficiently and effectively and may need to be practised/developed

➡ Admitting your concerns about any area of practice should not be considered a failure in your ability to practise but a strength in your professional development.

## Self-assessment questions

(?) What skills will you need to implement the care plan?

(?) How will you know if the care plan has been implemented properly?

(?) How can you develop your own skills to implement the care plan?

(?) What laws and/or policies influence how you record information?

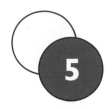

# 5 Evaluating the care plan

**This chapter will help you to:**
- ➡ Identify the importance of evaluation.
- ➡ Discuss the role of clinical and social governance in evaluation.
- ➡ Discuss the role of supervision in evaluation.
- ➡ Discuss accountability and empowerment of the practitioner in evaluating a care plan.

## Introduction

*Research is composed of many stories.*

(Church 1995: 9)

It would be easy to say that evaluation is the final stage in the care planning process, but in reality, as with the assessment stage, you will be evaluating all the time. It would be unethical not to make changes until the allocated evaluation date if you see that something is going wrong beforehand. There are many practical approaches to evaluation which are usually documented in the care plan, such as who needs to be informed and when the next evaluation meeting will be held, and these require organizational skills; however, there are other skills that will help you to evaluate more effectively and efficiently. These skills have been mentioned briefly in previous chapters but will be explored in more detail here. They will help you to develop personally and professionally and to feel empowered as being influential in the care planning process – just as influential as the person you are planning the care for. Without a feeling of empowerment, practitioners will quickly lose interest in delivering high quality care and their work will become 'just a job' (Hawkins and Shohet 2006). The QAA (2006: 6) suggest that practitioners should be able to:

- assess and document the outcomes of their practice;
- involve clients in assessing the effectiveness of the care given;
- learn from their practice to improve the care given in a particular case;
- learn from the experience to improve their future practice;
- participate in audit and other quality assurance procedures to contribute to effective risk management and good clinical governance;
- use the outcomes of evaluation to develop health and social care policy and practice.

# What is evaluation?

Evaluation is as much about the stories from your practice and the practice of your colleagues as it is about the care being delivered. This chapter will explore the stories that practitioners might bring to supervision about their practice informing the evaluation process. As previously identified, the care planning process is not a linear one but more of a spiral, where you may visit parts of the process many times over. It is rare if you are working with people with long-term conditions to go through the process only once as some people may take time to recover all or some of their independence. It is important therefore to check every so often to make sure that the care plan is still working in favour of the client and to make any adjustments as soon as possible.

---

**Hot topic**

The care plan is a legal document that can be used in a court of law. Consider what may be important areas for evaluation should you be required to submit any of your records to the courts. This is a useful exercise when casting an eye over your records during evaluation (e.g. has everything been signed and are all dates and signatures clear and legible?).

---

The evaluation stage involves informal as well as formal elements. Informal evaluation is also known as intuition, and is often frowned upon as being unprofessional. However, we cannot deny that we all experience intuition, and it would therefore be foolish to disregard its importance. Some authors refer to intuition as 'tacit' knowledge – unconscious knowledge that we do not know we have until we explore it through reflective practice and supervision (Ghaye 2000). Whether we call it tacit knowledge or intuition, it is what we do with this knowledge that is important. Intuition can be seen as an important part of the reflective/evaluative process, as it is usually some 'gut' feeling that alerts you to something not being quite right. Schön (1983) calls this 'reflecting on practice' and he also argues that practitioners are capable of reflecting while *in* practice.

---

**Practice point: informal/intuitive conversations**

You may be aware of people within your team chatting informally about care provision and individual clients. This informal discussion is often based on a hunch that something might need adjusting or is not going well. These discussions are just as important as formal evaluation and supervision but are often not documented. It is becoming more important for staff to document *all* discussions, however informal, so that evaluation processes can be tracked back and audited.

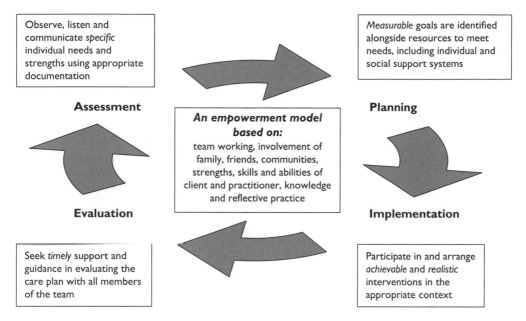

**Figure 5.1**  Evaluating the care plan using the empowerment model

Jaspers (2003) suggests that in order to develop our reflective skills we need to get to know ourselves, and it is useful to make a record of this from time to time. Using a SWOT analysis (A. Smith 2004) is usually a requisite of a practice portfolio to demonstrate self-understanding. However, it is amazing how many students and staff do not complete this process. A SWOT analysis may also be used to evaluate the effectiveness of your own practice and the care plan, and help the team to see where adjustments needs to be made.

A SWOT analysis is made up of the following components:

- *Strengths* – what are your strengths in this care plan? What do you think you have done well? You may find that you have good organizational and communication skills and that you are able to approach the rest of the team with confidence. This would lead to all the people involved in Brian's care having a good understanding of what is happening and would be evident in the smooth running of the care plan.

- *Weaknesses* – what are the weaknesses in this care plan and how are they identified? This does not necessarily mean they are *your* weaknesses but they may become evident as something you had not considered before implementing the care plan. Weaknesses are usually able to be strengthened once you have discovered what they are. For example, in the care plan for Brian you may have discovered that his appointments clashed so he was unable to attend one of them. This is easily remedied.

- *Opportunities* – what opportunities have presented themselves during the care planning process? For example, have you had the opportunity to learn more about what other members of the multidisciplinary team do, or to spend some time with individual practitioners? This may help you to gather information for Brian on how to manage his diabetes and you will be able to tell him more about the services available.
- *Threats* – what has threatened the care planning process? For example, you may find that the local transport system is unreliable or unavailable when Brian needs it, or that some practitioners are unable to see Brian quickly enough because they have a waiting list. If you are unable to do anything about these threats to Brian's care you must record them with your manager as *unmet needs*. This is important for clinical and social governance as it makes transparent where the needs of a local community are not being met and service developers can include these needs in their development plans.

## How to evaluate the care plan

Keeping track of the activities laid out in the care plan helps us to continually monitor the care given and make adjustments as required. This may occur on an informal or formal basis depending upon the original layout of the care plan and the wishes of the individual person. Sometimes we can put ourselves and the people we care for under too much pressure to achieve goals too soon, so it is important that the evaluation stage is agreed with the client and the care team. This will involve developing skills in managing the whole care planning process from assessment to evaluation in order to be able to lead other members of the team in caring for Brian. Remember that whatever you do as part of the evaluation process you must make sure it is documented.

### Time management

Evaluation may take place hourly, daily, weekly, monthly or at even greater intervals depending on the individual needs of the client and the resources available. Most areas of practice have a maximum time allowed for evaluation to take place and this will differ depending on the area of work (e.g. an intensive care ward may practise hourly evaluations). In the community it is recognized that more time may be needed to show signs of improvement and evaluation can take place, for example, every six months. However, it is important not to stick too rigidly to times and dates. If as the main practitioner you become aware that something has changed or is not quite right you are accountable to the patient and to your team to make sure people are aware of this and that it is addressed.

### Communication and organizational skills

Use the activity below to reflect on who is actually involved in Brian's care.

**Activity 5.1**

➡ Who are the main people involved in Brian's care?
➡ Who has an interest about whether the care interventions have been effective?
➡ Who are we as the care provider/coordinator accountable to for our practice under clinical/social and professional guidelines?

This is a useful activity to set yourself at frequent intervals outside the formal evaluation stage as it will help you to keep focused on your practice. You could use these questions as you reflect on your practice during your working day and in more formal supervision meetings.

All the communication skills that you have used throughout the process of care planning will need to be utilized to help you evaluate the care plan effectively. You will need to be able to competently listen to the concerns that people may have and guide them towards thinking about any other needs that may have arisen since the care plan was put into place. This will require a reassessment of any tools used to obtain measurement scores and to identify any improvements in Brian's health. Before an evaluation meeting, consider the following:

- Managing the environment – is there an appropriate place to meet, does everyone have transport, are there any specific needs for individuals (e.g. can Brian manage stairs)?
- Managing yourself – have you prepared yourself for the meeting by discussing and reflecting upon the care plan with your manager/supervisor and Brian?
- Managing the team – has the team identified any clinical/social governance issues that may need addressing?
- Obtaining information – this should be done in sufficient time for everyone (including Brian and his brother) to be able to read it and think about the questions they want to ask.

The empowerment model can help us to evaluate the care planning process, although the model may change if we are only providing a very specific part of the care plan. For example, the GP and practice nurse may use a biomedical model to evaluate their input into Brian's care plan which will enable them to focus more specifically on the biological aspects of his health needs in order to get his diabetes under control again.

## The client and person-centred care

Brian and his family must remain at the centre of the care planning process if it is to remain person-centred (Greenstreet 2006). Ultimately it is Brian who can tell us whether the care plan has been effective in meeting his needs (Kleinman 1988; Kitwood 1997; Lloyd 2009). We identified those needs in the assessment stage and we will need to evaluate each part of Brian's care plan that addresses those needs. We will have added dates in the evaluation column to remind us when we need to evaluate the care plan but this is not simply a matter of checking that everything is happening as it should: we will also need to see if the plan is working in helping Brian towards independence and recovery. As you can see from the completed care plan below, some needs will need to be evaluated weekly while others will take more time to address and can be evaluated monthly. Once a plan is established, some elements may be evaluated every six months or even once a year.

| Patient name    Brian Jones | | Date of birth    01/01/1955 | |
| --- | --- | --- | --- |
| *Needs* <br> (*specific: in person's own words where possible*) | *Goals* <br> (*measurable and achievable: including any assessment tool measurements*) | *Interventions* <br> (*realistic*) | *Evaluation* <br> (*timely*) |
| 1. Help with managing diabetes | **Short-term goal** <br> *To stabilize diabetes with the help of the practice nurse, dietician and GP* <br><br> **Long-term goal** <br> *For Brian to maintain a healthy diet that reduces fluctuations in blood sugar levels and attend regular appointments with services* | *1. Arrange regular appointments with GP/practice nurse in local surgery for close monitoring of blood sugar levels* <br><br> *2. Contact local diabetic support group and help Brian make initial visit* <br><br> *3. Provide information for Brian and his brother on self-care and any other support available* | *Weekly* |
| 2. Help with mobility | **Short-term goal** <br> *GP and physiotherapist to assess and alleviate reported pain levels, currently 6 out of 10* <br><br> **Long-term goal** <br> *For Brian to feel less pain on moving and to be able to attend meetings and socialize more frequently* | *1. Arrange appointment with doctor to discuss pain and treatment options* <br> *2. Help Brian to attend any outpatient appointments (e.g. pain clinic, diabetes clinic, physiotherapy, occupational therapy)* <br> *3. Arrange transport to help Brian attend appointments* | *Monthly* |

| | | | |
|---|---|---|---|
| 3. Low mood | **Short-term goal**<br>Care coordinator to provide and discuss information on how to manage the condition<br><br>**Long-term goal**<br>For Brian to be more in control of his life and his future | 1. Assess mood using specific tools<br>2. Obtain information on self-care and discuss with Brian<br>3. Help Brian to access information( e.g. via internet at local library)<br>4. Discuss with Brian options and risks when managing his condition<br>5. Discuss with Brian the benefits of keeping a mood diary | Monthly |
| 4. Sleep excess | **Short-term goal**<br>Care coordinator to assess and monitor sleep pattern<br><br>**Long-term goal**<br>For Brian to sleep less and have more time in the day to take care of himself | 1. Help Brian to identify his individual sleep pattern<br>2. Obtain information to help Brian improve his sleep pattern<br>3. Discuss with Brian the benefits of keeping a sleep diary | Weekly |
| 5. Lacks social support | **Short-term goal**<br>Social worker to increase access to social networks<br><br>**Long-term goal**<br>For Brian to have a wider support network to help him self-care by increasing contacts with other organizations/people | 1. Identify local support networks with Brian<br>2. Help Brian to choose which support networks to contact/attend<br>3. Help Brian to identify transport options<br>4. Help Brian to obtain financial support with transport costs where available | Monthly |
| **Signatures** | Care coordinator<br>A.N. Other, RN | Client<br>Brian Jones | Date<br>01/02/10 |

## Practitioner involvement and supervision

When looking at the care plan you can see that there are many stakeholders involved and you might think that the care coordinator does not do a great deal to help Brian in meeting his health and social care needs. However, the coordinator is the linchpin that holds the whole care plan together (Allison 2005; Firth-Cozens and Cornwell 2009). It is very important therefore that the care coordinator is aware of their own values and practices and how they have influenced the planning process. One way of developing such awareness is through refection, which was discussed in the previous chapter.

---

**Hot topic**

How can we be sure that we have addressed all of Brian's needs? You may want to discuss this with your manager or supervisor and document your discussion in Brian's notes. One way of doing this is by reflecting on what assessments have been carried out with Brian to help him identify his needs – can you name them? This will provide evidence that you have done your best to address all of Brian's needs.

---

If we refer back to the EVENT framework in Chapter 4 we can add another letter to the process: 'S' for supervision, giving the acronym EVENTS. Supervision is a good way of talking over your concerns and beliefs with someone who you value for their experience and honesty and who can help you to develop your skills. Hawkins and Shohet (2006: 3) state that in times of stress supervision is extremely important. They support this suggestion by adding:

> it can give us a chance to stand back and reflect; a chance to avoid the easy way out by blaming others – clients, peers, the organization, society or even oneself; and it can give us the chance to search for new options, to discover the learning that often emerges from the most difficult situations and to get support.

It is advisable to have had at least one supervision meeting regarding Brian's care plan before it is evaluated but if you are at all concerned about any aspect of a person's care plan you should seek supervision immediately if you are unable to manage the situation or risk. There is no excuse for not acting even if it is a simple phone call that you later document as having taken place to demonstrate that you did not ignore a situation. Most people would prefer that you checked something out with them, whether they be the client or your manager, rather than say nothing and hope that a problem will go away.

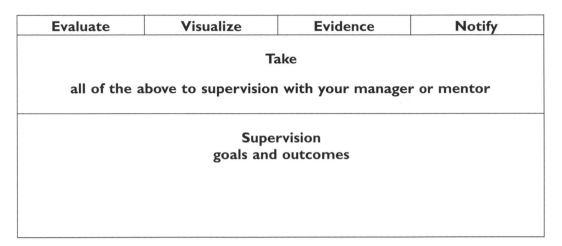

| Evaluate | Visualize | Evidence | Notify |
|----------|-----------|----------|--------|
| **Take** | | | |
| **all of the above to supervision with your manager or mentor** | | | |
| **Supervision goals and outcomes** | | | |

**Figure 5.2**  EVENTS framework for reflective practice and supervision meetings

Supervision is good practice because although you are already reflecting upon an event you may not be sure whether the outcome is the one that you should have expected. This is where reflective practice can actually let practitioners down because, as Ghaye (2000) suggests, there needs to be a reflective conversation taking place for it to be effective. Always take your reflective practice notes to your supervision meetings for discussion. By doing this you will have feedback from someone who can help you develop and broaden your perspective on the quality agenda and consequently the care planning process.

---

**Practice point: the supervision process**

Different organizations will have different policies regarding practice supervision, which should be different to management supervision. However, this is not always clear to practitioners except in that they have usually been told that supervision is supported in the workplace. Practitioners may then wait for it to be given rather than seeking a supervisor out. If you are allocated a supervisor make sure you have regular meetings with them and preferably a contract (which may look similar to a care plan of your own).

---

We will now expand our reflection on Brian's care to include the outcomes from supervision with a mentor or tutor.

| Evaluate | Visualize | Evidence | Notify |
|---|---|---|---|
| Brian did not attend an appointment | Need to review transport arrangements for appointments | Poor mobility may be making it difficult for Brian to access services | Let the team know that transport/access is presenting a problem |

**Take**
**all of the above to supervision with your manager or mentor**

*Discuss in supervision the following:*

*How to help Brian gain better access to services*

*What has been discussed with Brian and how he thinks this issue can be improved*

**Supervision goals and outcomes**

- *Care coordinator to explore with Brian alternative transport arrangements*
- *Care coordinator to discuss with the team how appointments can be better organized*
- *Care coordinator to review with Brian whether his mobility had improved and if there are any other needs relating to this part of the care plan*
- *Care coordinator to document in care record the outcomes of supervision*

**Figure 5.3** EVENTS framework for reflective practice and supervision goals

## Team involvement

It may often seem to the practitioner that they are alone in delivering the care plan, but if this becomes strongly evident then it is even more important to call a team meeting of all those involved. This will help to improve the quality of care and reduce burnout and stress among staff by opening up communication channels.

Members of the multidisciplinary team involved in Brian's care are:

- the care coordinator – organizing the care plan and providing information;
- the GP and practice nurse – monitoring blood levels and diet;
- the social worker – accessing wider support networks and transport;
- the consultant and physiotherapist – monitoring physical health and mobility needs;
- voluntary organizations and local community – providing support and self-care advice;
- Brian's brother, who also acts as an informal carer.

In order to evaluate the care provided, you and Brian will need to talk to all of these people to gather their opinion on whether they have seen any improvement and whether they have any suggestions for future care provision. This could be carried out on an individual basis, but most teams prefer where possible to come together for a formally recorded meeting. This can be sometimes difficult to arrange but if it is achievable it will be invaluable for all concerned.

## Carer involvement

Here is an extract from a carer's evaluation of the care planning process.

> *Well, when she was in the hospital ... a social worker who was ... from the hospital contacted me. Now I thought she was an NHS worker. No one ... had explained to me that she was a Social Services social worker with an office at the hospital to look after the patients' interests in that hospital. And when my wife then went into the residential home, I contacted her with a query one day and she said, 'Oh I'm not your wife's social worker any more, she, the social worker is now ... and you'll contact her at the Social Services office.' But no one had explained, I was a bit baffled by all this. It all seemed very confusing. I didn't realise, no one said, 'Well I only look after the interests of patients here.' I would have understood then straight away. Those are the kind of things that leave you a little bit confused in the beginning.*

You can read the whole transcript at www.healthtalkonline.org/Nerves_and_Brian/Carers_of_people_with_dementia/Topic/2118/Interview/665/Clip/3790.

Carers may be providing a large part of the care that would otherwise require a hospital stay or intense home care. They are valued members of the team and the care plan may well depend on them in their role as carer for the client. However, the needs of the carer often go unnoticed, which can lead to their own health deteriorating as a result. Loss of income, social support and healthy lifestyle can lead to such deterioration very quickly if not identified. Carers have for some time been entitled to an assessment and a care plan of their own if necessary under the Carer and Disabled Children Act 2000, and are also entitled under the Human Rights Act 1998 and the Carers Equal Opportunities Act 2004 to have access to work and education if required. The relationship between Brian and his brother is important to Brian and it should therefore be evident in Brian's notes that an assessment and, if required, a care plan be offered to his brother.

---

**Activity 5.2**

If we were to carry out an assessment of Brian's brother, what might his needs be? You can use the same assessment tools as those for Brian to make sure you have holistically assessed his brother's needs including:

- Physical
- Psychological
- Social
- Spiritual

---

## The organization

Through regular case note audit the organization has a requirement on its entire staff to provide information on all areas of clinical and social governance. This includes the outcomes of the care planning process which can only be identified through a formal evaluation. However, the evaluation process is not the same as a case note audit and should not be seen as a 'tick box' exercise. This stage of the care planning framework will result in three main outcomes:

❶ The care plan is no longer needed and Brian is completely self-managing his diabetes and social needs.
❷ The care plan needs to be changed to accommodate new needs/information.
❸ The care plan should stay the same.

The importance of managing long-term conditions is not to save money and refuse care to people but to ensure that every person with a long-term condition is getting the right care at the right time (DoH 2005a, 2005b). Without evaluation processes we would have no way of knowing if this was the case. We do know however that as people are living longer there will be an increased need for patients with long-term conditions to have a care plan that is SMART and effective in meeting the quality agenda of health and social care.

In Chapter 7 the quality agenda will be discussed in more detail together with the roles and responsibilities of the different organizations. Ultimately every person's role within an organization is to provide the best possible individualized care and this has become more evident in the policy documents that have emerged in recent years. It is important to remember that it is everyone's responsibility at every level to provide good quality care and this should not just be the responsibility of our managers or those in more senior positions to us.

---

**Hot topic**

The legal system is an area of practice often overlooked in health care more than social care but we must be mindful of how this system affects what we do and how we do it. Try to reflect on how many laws affect your day-to-day practice and what influence they might have.

---

Figure 5.4 will help you to reflect on the quality of the care plan for Brian and whether there are areas for improvement from an individual practitioner point of view and/or an organizational point of view. While a 'tick box' approach to evaluation is not recommended, having a checklist to refer back to will help you to expand on the client's, team's and organization's narrative. How many of the following could you discuss as being identified within Brian's care plan?

| Identifying and managing risk | Public and patient involvement (PPI) at the strategic and individual level | Regular clinical and/or social audit |
|---|---|---|
| Gathering information on the patient/client experience | **Clinical and social governance agenda/areas of inspection** | Evidence-based practice |
| Strategic capacity and resource management | Making use of information technology | Staffing management and CPD |

**Figure 5.4**  Key areas of the clinical and social governance agenda (adapted from DoH 1997 and SCIE 2007)

## Duty of care

When evaluating a care plan and its outcomes it is important to establish whether the practitioners concerned have successfully met their *duty of care*. We have a duty of care to ensure that we are doing all that we can for Brian. If one of the following events occurred, would it constitute a failure of our duty of care?

- failing to visit Brian without letting him know;
- failing to contact his GP or practice nurse to make sure his blood sugar levels are acceptable;
- taking Brian to a football match instead of an appointment with the consultant;
- leaving lots of information with Brian for him to read at his leisure.

All of the above are risks to Brian's health. Some of them are obviously neglectful (e.g. failing to visit Brian). Taking him to a football match at his request in itself can be seen as a positive step in terms of his socialization, but should not have taken place at the expense of a hospital appointment with the consultant. The health and social care workers union Unison (2003: 13) provide a very useful handbook, free to download, that examines an employee's duty of care in some detail. In essence however, employees must exercise a duty of care:

- to patients;
- to colleagues;
- to themselves.

A skilled person (i.e. a medical professional) who has a duty of care must:

- keep their knowledge up to date;

- provide a good quality service;
- be able to identify risks;
- keep a record of all activity;
- only delegate or be delegated to when sure that competence can be maintained;
- respect confidentiality unless it is in the best interests of the person to share information.

A duty of care protects the individual from negligent acts which can be proved to be harmful in some way. In the evaluation stage therefore we need to be able to provide evidence that Brian has received the best possible care.

---

**Activity 5.3**

You were asked to consider the above list of actions in relation to Brian's care and whether they could be deemed negligent. Some of the answers may not have been evident but in general any act of omission (i.e. not doing something) could be seen as negligent. Abuse is another area of practice that may occur unknowingly (but may still be classed as an offence) and you may need to think carefully about some interactions with clients identified by Kitwood (1997) and discussed in Chapters 1 and 2.

---

The following example shows how you might write up an evaluation meeting. Remember to keep it as short as possible, keep to the facts and keep it SMART.

**Checklist for care planning audit**

| Date | Record to be made at least once daily or on every contact | Signature and designation |
|------|-----------------------------------------------------------|---------------------------|
| 01/02/10 | *Brian's care plan was reviewed today in a multidisciplinary team meeting held at the Team Base at 2 p.m. All members of the team attended except the GP who gave his apologies, however the practice nurse attended on his behalf. The team agreed that the care plan was working very well and Brian and his brother had no general comments and had discussed the care plan previously with myself the care coordinator as follows:* <br><br> ***1. Help with diabetes*** <br> *It was agreed that the need to visit the GP surgery every week was no longer necessary as Brian's blood sugar levels were becoming stable again and he could attend on a monthly basis instead. Brian and his brother were satisfied with the support provided by the local voluntary group and were in weekly contact with them.* | *A.N. Other, RN* |

*expected    outcomes*

**2. Help with mobility**
*Brian reported that his pain level had reduced from 6 to 4 and he was having regular monthly appointments with his consultant and/or physiotherapist.*

**3. Low mood**
*Brian's mood had improved and he was feeling more hopeful about his future and making plans to develop his own interests.*

**4. Excessive sleep**
*Brian was now in a regular sleep pattern and averaging eight hours of unbroken sleep per night.*

**5. Lack of social support**
*Brian was now attending an art class once a week and going out with his brother once a week to shop for food, which he felt was enough activity for his current mobility levels.*

*Brian did raise the issue of costs in regard to travelling and said he was finding it difficult to afford public transport and a good diet. It was agreed that his social worker would explore his eligibility for a free bus pass and whether he could claim direct payments to attend the art class as these were effectively a service that he was purchasing himself.*

**6. Date of next review**
*It was agreed to review the care plan in six months.*

The new care plan would now be rewritten with adjustments made to the number of needs that were outstanding or at risk, and therefore required further interventions. The care plan would then look more like this example and would be distributed to everyone involved to inform them of the changes as soon as possible.

| Patient Name    Brian Jones | | Date of Birth    01/01/1955 | |
|---|---|---|---|
| **Needs** <br> (*specific: in person's own words where possible*) | **Goals** <br> (*measurable and achievable: including any assessment tool measurements*) | **Interventions** <br> (*realistic*) | **Evaluation** <br> (*timely*) |
| *1. Help with managing diabetes* | **Short-term goal** <br> *To stabilize diabetes with the help of doctor, practice nurse and dietician* <br><br> **Long-term goal** <br> *For Brian to maintain a healthy diet that reduces fluctuations in blood sugar levels* | *1. Arrange monthly appointments with GP/practice nurse in local surgery for close monitoring of blood sugar levels* | *Six months* |
| *2. Help with mobility* | **Short-term goal** <br> *Doctor and physiotherapist to assess and alleviate reported pain levels – 6 out of 10 baseline assessment (4 out of 10 at one-month review)* <br><br> **Long-term goal** <br> *For Brian to feel less pain when moving and to be able to attend appointments/ meetings more easily* | *1. Social worker to help Brian access free bus pass/transport* | *Six months* |
| *3. Lacks social support* | **Short-term goal** <br> *Social worker to help Brian increase access to social networks* <br><br> **Long-term goal** <br> *For Brian to have a wider support network to help him self-care by increasing contacts with other organizations/people* | *1. Social worker to help Brian to obtain financial support with accessing art group where available* | *Six months* |
| **Signatures** | Care coordinator <br><br> A.N. Other, RN | Client <br><br> Brian Jones | Date <br><br> 01/02/10 |

## Chapter summary

➡ The evaluation stage is an important part of the care planning process and helps us to measure progress and/or risk.

➡ Practice supervision is a place to discuss our concerns and practice with a qualified practitioner.

➡ We all have a duty of care to our clients, colleagues and employers.

➡ Neglect (and abuse) may occur when we have not thought through why we are taking or not taking certain actions with a client.

## Self-assessment questions

❓ How will I know when to evaluate part of, or the entire, care plan?

❓ Who can I go to for help?

❓ How can I ensure all of the multidisciplinary team has been involved in evaluating the care plan?

❓ How can I identify my own learning needs?

# 6 Revisiting the care planning process

**This chapter will help you to:**

➡ Summarize the care planning process.
➡ Identify significant components of care planning.
➡ Discuss practitioner knowledge and skills.
➡ Make recommendations for future care planning practice.

## Introduction

*A narrative can be understood to organise a sequence of events into a whole so that the significance of each event can be understood through its relation to that whole. In this way a narrative conveys the meaning of events.*

(Elliott 2005 :3)

It may come as no surprise that while this book has been in production, and no doubt after it has been published, social policy and law will continue to drive health and social care forward with more and more guidelines and policies which each individual working in different areas of practice must try to keep up with. Indeed, the Health and Social Care Act 2008 heralds major changes in how health and social care is inspected and audited for evidence of good quality care provision (see Chapter 7). However, many practitioners who are already working in the health and social care field know that the philosophies, principles and processes of health and social care have remained fairly consistent over the last decade and match the main principles of the empowerment model of care planning that recognizes the importance of person-centred care and a 'whole-system' approach. This is where the client's narrative becomes visible in identifying what has happened to address their needs and how the care plan has facilitated this. All your hard work in assessing, planning, implementing and evaluating the care plan could appear wasted if the individual or team does not agree with it. Therefore, compromise and negotiation must be recognized as successful drivers of any care plan. Good interpersonal and reflective skills are an essential requirement of the process in order to ensure that the person receives the best possible care. This chapter will evaluate the narrative of events in planning care for and with Brian and, like a good care plan, make recommendations for future implementation in practice.

## Focusing on the quality agenda: key recommendations

By now it is hoped that you will have a better understanding of the quality agenda and how it can help us to provide good quality care. When writing care plans it becomes more and more obvious that this is a skill that once learned will become transferable to many patients with different needs.

Social and clinical governance agendas have made quite clear the areas of practice for which we are all responsible to some degree or another. This may differ depending upon our roles and responsibilities, but an awareness of the whole quality agenda will help us to put our own practice into perspective. With the help of our fictitious client, Brian, we can now explore the quality agenda in relation to his care plan. By bringing together policy, law and person-centred practice we can ensure that we have addressed the needs of the organization as well as the person who is seeking help from that organization. This whole-systems approach (DoH 2003d) will then lead us to some key recommendations for future practice that will empower both the client and the practitioner to make best use of the information, knowledge and skills that they both share.

---

**Activity 6.1**

Look at the health and social care governance agenda in Figure 6.1 and consider how the various elements relate to Brian's individual care plan (this could be used as a quick checklist for other care plans too). Then read on for the answers.

---

| Identifying and managing risk | Public and patient involvement (PPI) at the strategic and individual level | Regular clinical and/or social audit |
|---|---|---|
| Gathering information on the patient/client experience | **Clinical and social governance agenda/areas of inspection** | Evidence-based practice |
| Strategic capacity and resource management | Making use of information technology | Staffing management and CPD |

**Figure 6.1**  Key areas of the clinical and social governance agenda (adapted from DoH 1997 and SCIE 2007)

Key recommendation 1: identifying and managing risk

Brian's health was at risk because his diabetes was unstable and so this needed to be a high priority within the care plan. Helping Brian to keep in regular contact with his GP practice enabled him to discuss the day-to-day management of his diabetes. He was also referred to a consultant who could make further investigations into why Brian's diabetes had become unstable. Because of his long-term illness Brian was also at risk of losing contact with his friends and brother and was in danger of suffering from depression if he was not empowered to regain control of his life. Risks and needs are often linked, because each need can present a risk if not properly addressed. This is where positive risk-taking becomes important. The DoH (2007a: 50) has produced a checklist to help practitioners and clients address risks within a care plan which covers:

- *Dignity* – have the person's feelings concerning what might happen to them been identified and addressed and has their personhood been maintained?
- *Diversity* – have the person's different or unique needs been identified and addressed?
- *Religious and spiritual needs* – does the person need to carry out regular worship or rituals and have these needs been identified and addressed?
- *Personal strengths* – have the person's skills been identified and included in the assessment?
- *Ability and willingness to be supported to self-care* – how willing is the person to work towards self-care?
- *Opportunities to learn new skills* – is education and information available for the person to develop new skills?
- *Support networks* – are there local support networks available to help the person meet their needs?
- *Information needs* – has all the information been provided in a manner that is acceptable to the person (e.g. face-to-face contact, written material, electronic links to audio and visual material)?
- *Communication needs* – does the person have needs in terms of their communication skills (e.g. reading, writing or language)?
- *Environment* – is the environment suitable and safe for addressing health and social care needs?
- *Ability to identify own risks* – is the person able to notify others when risks become evident and do they have access to a means of fast communication (e.g. telephone, email or mobile phone)?
- *Ability to find solutions* – is the person able to identify and offer preferred choices in managing risk?
- *Social isolation, inclusion and exclusion* – does the local community include or exclude certain groups of people (e.g. older people)?
- *Least restrictive options* – have all options been provided so that the least restrictive can be chosen?

- *Quality of life outcomes and risk to independence of 'not supporting choice'* – have these outcomes or risks been made clear to the person but without threat so that they may choose a more harmful option if they wish?

In Brian's assessment we identified the risks shown in the general risk assessment below, which were incorporated into his care plan. Many of the above issues can be found in Brian's risk assessment. However, without drawing too much attention to the risks themselves, we took a whole-person approach to incorporating them into the care plan and addressing Brian's needs. Some care planning documentation keeps the risk assessment and interventions separate from the main care plan but this runs the risk of them becoming detached and lost, or simply ignored altogether. The important thing to remember is to identify as many risks as possible and document how they will be addressed. Simply carrying out a risk assessment and then doing nothing is of no use to anyone at all.

The QAA (2006: 4) health and social care benchmark statement suggests that it is the responsibility of the practitioner to manage risk as follows:

*Health and social care staff should:*

- *act properly to protect clients, patients, the public and colleagues from the risk of harm*
- *ensure that their own or their colleagues' health, conduct or performance does not place clients and patients at risk*
- *protect clients and patients from risks of infection or other dangers in the environment*

Risk assessment should therefore be taken in the broadest sense without leaving anything out that we think may affect the care provided for Brian, and include environmental as well as individual factors. Brian identified how he had tried to manage the risks and we were able to help him find other ways of managing these risks via regular appointments with experts who could advise him.

## General risk assessment

| Area of risk | Current needs | Positive risks taken |
|---|---|---|
| Hypothermia | No | |
| Neglect | Diet sometimes neglected | Brother helps me sometimes |
| Abuse, physical, emotional, financial | No | |
| Exploitation | No | |

| | | |
|---|---|---|
| Slips, trips and falls | Pain in legs sometimes makes me fall | Use furniture in house and walking stick outside |
| Isolation | Retired so not very sociable | None |
| Nutrition and hydration | Sometimes eat wrong foods for diabetes | Talk to doctor about it sometimes |
| Suicide/self-harm | Wonder what's the point sometimes | Not good at talking to people |
| Violence/aggression | No | |

## Key recommendation 2: public/patient involvement

The government has introduced Public and Patient Involvement (PPI) and Local Involvement Network forums (LINks) to ensure that all health and social care organizations consult with the local public on local needs. The *Health Select Committee Inquiry into Patient and Public Involvement in the NHS* (DoH 2007b) suggests that PPI is difficult to define because it covers such a wide range of patient activities which may include some or all of the following:

- participation in treatment decisions with the clinician;
- exercising choice over which hospital or GP to use;
- giving their views on specific services;
- giving their views on specific policy developments;
- joining a group that provides advice to organizations and trusts;
- participating in national consultations;
- exercising their voting rights to choose political leaders.

It is easy to see how this can cause confusion for service providers as well as people who use those services. Some organizations are good at participation in some of the above but not all, and it needs to be made clear to staff and clients what level of involvement is required and being applied. Most people now agree that those who suffer from long-term conditions are 'experts by experience' and together with more professional expertise can improve service delivery and outcomes. (For more information on the 'Expert Patients Programme' see DoH 2001b: 5.) The following is an excerpt from that document on why patient involvement is important:

> *The experiences of people with chronic diseases in using health services are very variable. In the better services people are given advice and information and their questions are answered. But few go beyond this to ensure that a patient's growing knowledge of his or her condition is developed to a level whereby self-management, within the boundaries of a medical regime, becomes a real option. The impact of this*

*has been considerable. Individuals have experienced unnecessary pain and discomfort along with a severe limitation to their quality of life. There is also an economic cost to society from avoidable absence from work and inflated health and social services costs.*

Brian was involved in his care plan and was invited to outline his needs in his own words. This helped everyone to see Brian's perspective and how he would like help with certain aspects of his life. Brian was not incapacitated by his illness and was therefore able to make all the decisions himself. However, we did consider that if he were unconscious and/or unable to make decisions then we would need to act in his best interests under the Mental Capacity Act 2005.

Continued consultation with Brian took place as part of the evaluation stage when we asked him how he thought his care plan had been working. He identified a problem that was overlooked by the professional team, which was a lack of finances to access and attend appointments, leisure groups etc. This could have caused the care plan to fail if not addressed, as Brian would not have had the money to carry out his care plan. It is easy to assume that we have covered everything, especially if we think we have an in-depth knowledge of an area of practice; however, it is often the little things that may be overlooked such as sufficient funds, budgeting skills or an impaired ability to read or hear what is being said that cause care plans to fail. If we do not involve the client in their care plan they will be unable to tell us when it is not working. In order to take action quickly when things go wrong we need the client's input into the monitoring and evaluation as much as anyone else's, so that we can advocate on their behalf.

---

**Practice point: duty to involve**

Under the Health and Social Care Act 2008 both local authorities and the NHS have a duty to involve clients by listening to their experiences and inviting them to take part in developing new services. In your own area of practice, do you know how clients are involved in developing your service?

---

## Key recommendation 3: regular audit

It was identified as we worked through the care planning process why it is important to keep up-to-date records of everything that we do so that our managers can audit the process. This is especially important when something is not going right but should always be carried out so that a history of interventions can be produced. It is also a requirement of our professional and educational standards that we can evidence our actions at all times. The following checklist outlines much of what has been identified in this book and will help you check your care planning records. It could also be used for auditing purposes unless there are more service-centred auditing tools available. Many audit documents will look similar to the one below. They are also often included at the back of social policy documents such as *Adult Mental Health Services, Stronger in*

*Partnership 2: Involving Service Users and Carers in the Design, Planning, Delivery and Evaluation of Mental Health Services in Wales* (Welsh Assembly Government 2008). Page 5 of these guidelines suggests that 'Client involvement should not be seen as a one off intervention or a discrete piece of work; rather, it should be seen far more broadly as a more empowering way of working that needs to be an integral part of every aspect of mental health design, commissioning and provision'.

### Checklist for care planning audit

| Evidence | Location in records (or noted for improvement and underlined) | Date and signature |
|---|---|---|
| Philosophy of care followed or professional codes/values adhered to | | |
| All paperwork signed and dated | | |
| Good record-keeping practices (e.g. factual, timely, non-judgemental, client involvement, jargon-free, SMART) | | |
| Initial assessment containing basic personal information, regularly updated | | |
| Full holistic assessment completed | | |
| Models and/or frameworks used | | |
| Risk assessment completed and updated at evaluation | | |
| Health and safety issues identified | | |

| | | |
|---|---|---|
| Client's own words used | | |
| Client's needs identified | | |
| Reflection upon practice | | |
| National Service Frameworks followed | | |
| Evidenced-based practice | | |
| Social policy/guidance followed | | |
| Application of relevant laws (e.g. Mental Capacity Act) | | |
| Personal and professional development identified | | |
| Team/multidisciplinary working | | |
| Resource allocation | | |
| Environmental and/or cultural needs identified | | |
| Other (specific to individual workplace) | | |

## Key recommendation 4: evidence-based practice

It was highlighted in Chapter 3 why it is important to know how to find the evidence for our practice and how we might use that evidence to make sure we are advocating the best possible care for Brian. In this instance National Service Frameworks are available for diabetes so we can check if we are following all the correct procedures for Brian and establish that five out of the nine National Service Frameworks for people who suffer from diabetes (DoH 2001a: 5) have been met while the other four are not relevant to his individual needs at this time. These five are shown below in bold and this demonstrates that our care plan for Brian is meeting quality audit requirements.

- Prevention of Type 2 diabetes (which is also known as late onset or diet controlled diabetes).
- **Identification of people with diabetes (including those who do not know they have diabetes).**
- **Empowering people with diabetes in decision-making and maintaining healthy lifestyles.**
- **Clinical care of adults with diabetes.**
- Clinical care of children and young people with diabetes.
- **Management of diabetic emergencies.**
- Care of people with diabetes during admission to hospital.
- Diabetes and pregnancy.
- **Detection and management of long-term complications.**

---

**Hot topic**

National Service Frameworks now shape our policies and everyday practice. It may be worth taking some time to think about what policies and frameworks affect your practice and whether they are founded in evidence-based practice. Some policies, although official, can have very little evidence to support them, so it is important as a practitioner to be able to see where, in your own area of practice, there is strong evidence to support what you do.

---

For Brian we were not expected to know all about diabetes but we needed to know how to access further help for him in terms of his particular needs. This is where multidisciplinary team working is most effective in that people who do have more knowledge can become involved. Brian had the benefit of the expertise and knowledge of his GP, the practice nurse, a consultant and a physiotherapist who together helped him regain control over his health and physical activity. Team-working skills are very important for effective care coordination as there will need to be a lot of communication and information-sharing between the team members.

## Key recommendation 5: staffing management and CPD

While we may not all have the responsibility of managing other staff we do have a responsibility for our own developmental needs. Chapter 5 discussed how these might be addressed in practice supervision and how many of our professional codes of conduct require us to make it known to our managers if we feel unable to carry out an intervention. The EVENTS framework has been developed within this book to help you keep on track of your own personal and professional development needs.

Staff needs are just as important as the client's needs because without your needs being met you will be unable to do your job properly and effectively. Identifying staff needs may be carried out in a variety of ways and will include individual and group meetings. If staff within health and social care organizations are expected to work as teams in providing care then there are also issues within each team that will need addressing and acting upon. This is where your manager will play an important role in making sure everyone feels part of the team and feels as if they have been listened to. Hawkins and Shohet (2006) suggest that practice supervisors may have a variety of roles such as:

- a counsellor, offering support at stressful times;
- an educator, guiding people towards extending their learning and knowledge;
- a manager, responsible for the quality of work carried out with clients;
- a practitioner, with responsibilities to the organization and the team in which they themselves work.

A lack of team cohesion will quickly result in communication breakdown, which must be avoided at all costs as it can have very serious repercussions. The effectiveness of the whole team has a direct influence on the quality of care provided and a team needs constant support to maintain good quality care. It was identified in Chapter 3 how effective partnership working can contribute to good quality care planning (Allison 2005). Good partnership working involves:

- *candour* – awareness of confidentiality is maintained in supervision;
- *competence* – can be identified as a 'practitioner developmental need' in supervision;
- *diligence* – changes in the care plan or client needs can be discussed in supervision;
- *loyalty* – to the person in need of our help and to our employers, managers and the rest of the team;
- *fairness* – including non-discriminatory practice;
- *discretion* – about how much and what information needs to be shared.

Some teams will dedicate certain days during the year to review their practices and set some ground rules so that they are all aware of the function and roles of the team. However, this will depend on the type of team you are working in and whether you are all in regular daily contact or meet on a less frequent basis. The QAA (2006: 4) identifies the importance of team working and the educational development of staff in the following sections:

### 1.6 Cooperation and collaboration with colleagues

*Health and social care staff should:*

- *Respect and encourage the skills and contributions which colleagues in both their own profession and other professions bring to the care of clients and patients*
- *Within their work environment, support colleagues to develop their professional knowledge, skills and performance*
- *Not require colleagues to take on responsibilities that are beyond their level of knowledge, skills and experience.*

### 1.7 Education

*Health and social care staff should, where appropriate:*

- *Contribute to the education of students, colleagues, clients and patients, and the wider public*
- *Develop skills of responsible and proper supervision.*

There are expectations therefore upon practitioners to not only take care of themselves and their individual learning needs but also those of the team in which they work. Many teams develop social activities as a way of helping individuals to get to know each other better in a less formal setting outside work.

## Key recommendation 6: making use of information technology

The time will soon be upon us when all record-keeping and case notes will be electronic and we will all need to be able to communicate electronically. This is more difficult than face-to-face conversation as we cannot assume that other people have understood what we are trying to say when we write something down. It is important therefore to stick to the facts only, avoid making jokes and to remember to be SMART in every part of the care plan. We are already using the internet to access information but we need to be able to identify what information is reliable as evidence-based practice and what is not. Information technology is also a way of obtaining evidence for our practice quickly, whether from research or policy and legal documents. Many of the documents used in this book have links in the reference section to their electronic source.

Some staff have a fear of using the internet or simply refuse or lack the skills to do so, but remember that if you are following your professional codes of conduct then it is your responsibility to take action to keep your knowledge base up to date. If information is only (or more easily) available online and you make no attempt to access it, then you may be found to be an incompetent practitioner in the future.

Information technology covers a wide area of our everyday lives and can lead to a blurring of the boundaries between our personal and professional lives. There are many ways to communicate via the internet now that were not available a few years ago and this requires an awareness and understanding of how communicating electronically can differ from communicating verbally. This is known as *netiquette* and some useful tips on communicating in this way can be found on dedicated websites such as www.albion.com/netiquette.

### Tips for electronic communication

- Be very careful about making jokes on the internet: the other person cannot see if you are smiling or laughing.
- Be careful to whom you reply, make sure that you do not choose the 'reply all' button if you only want to reply to one person.
- Do not reply to any messages in an emotional or intoxicated state as you may regret it when you are in a more reasonable state.
- Always remember, once you hit the 'send' button your communication has gone and you cannot get it back.

Key recommendation 7: strategic capacity and resource management

Many of us may think that this is a management task, but managers are unable to manage resources without us keeping them informed of what is needed and what is not. If at any stage we are unable to access the resources identified in Brian's care plan we have a duty to report this to our managers as soon as possible. If we do not do so we could be increasing the risk of Brian's health deteriorating and could be found guilty of neglect. We are also duty-bound by the Health and Safety at Work Act 1974, which outlines the duties that employers have to staff, clients and carers and also the duties employees have to their managers and members of the public.

This means that whenever we identify from a risk assessment or other observation anything that could cause harm to those around us we have a duty to report it to our managers, preferably in writing so that there is a record. Whatever the manager decides to do with that information is then their responsibility but if we have not reported a concern and put it in writing then there is no evidence that it has been identified and/or addressed. However, in everyday practice it is not always so easy to identify health and safety risks and many practices are just accepted as being part of the job. Consider the following fairly common scenarios and think about your responsibility in relation to them in terms of health and safety:

- a client who refuses to take care of their personal hygiene;
- a colleague who arrives at work smelling of alcohol;
- a shortage of prescribed medication;
- a broken switch/plug/fitting;
- liquid on the floor;
- Christmas decorations on staircases;
- an aggressive pet;
- clients who smoke in their own homes;
- lone working;
- staff shortages.

There are probably many more you could add to this list but the important thing to remember is that they should all be reported to your manager/supervisor/mentor and a record should be made of what steps have been taken to remedy the situation.

Key recommendation 8: gathering information on the patient/client experience

The QAA (2006: 4) recognizes that clients have a right to be part of the evaluation process and that their contribution can affect the overall quality of care provided. However, it is the practitioner's responsibility to make sure that the client's views are heard and taken into account and to do this they should demonstrate the following values in their everyday practice:

- *be open and honest with clients and patients;*
- *listen to clients and patients;*

- *keep information about clients and patients confidential within the limits of duty of care;*
- *ensure that their own beliefs do not prejudice the care of their clients and patients;*
- *recognize and value cultural and social diversity;*
- *ensure individualized care and treatment to combat discrimination and social exclusion.*

Many of the above were identified in Chapter 2 which explored the assessment part of the care planning process. It was identified in that chapter how it was important to develop a therapeutic relationship with Brian so that his individual needs could be identified and addressed. Brian had self-managed his diabetes for many years but a change in social circumstances (retirement from his work) led to him losing touch with his individual needs. The assessment stage allowed practitioners to spend time with Brian and listen to his concerns. Good communication skills were necessary to identify, clarify and understand what Brian needed to help him regain his independence. The QAA (2006: 4) go on to suggest that health and social care staff should:

- *provide information about clients' and patients' health and social care options in a manner in which the clients and patients can understand;*
- *gain appropriate consent before giving care and treatment;*
- *enable clients and patients to make informed choices about care, including cases where those choices may result in adverse outcomes for the individual;*
- *provide clients and patients with proper access to their health and social care records.*

As practitioners we need to take a much wider view of the care planning process if we are to make sure that we are taking an empowering approach. This means that while we respect the needs of the individual we will also need to respect the community and the culture in which they live. For Brian, living in a rural village community meant that transport was not very reliable and this needed to be explored further. Brian also had a small support network consisting mainly of his brother's family which was widened to include local groups and activities.

## The empowerment model in practice

Now consider Figure 6.2. You can see how the empowerment model helps us to address many of the above quality agenda items.

How the empowerment model has helped us to address Brian's needs

- *Policy and law* were identified to help you understand why some areas are so important that there is a duty upon us to provide evidence that they have been attended to.
- *Local groups and voluntary organizations* were identified as helping Brian to extend his social network and providing specific advice and support in relation to his diabetes.

| Health and social care public policy and law (e.g. Mental Capacity Act 2005) | **Physical needs** Life skills Health skills Self-regulatory skills | Lobbying, advocacy and mediation from local groups (e.g. voluntary organizations) |
| --- | --- | --- |
| **Psychological needs** Reframing and adjustment of personal beliefs and attitudes | **The individual person** | **Social needs** Relationships and community empowerment including families, teams and services |
| Social, economic and environmental issues identified and addressed (e.g. access to health and social care, public transport etc.) | **Spiritual needs** Locus of control Self-efficacy Health literacy | Critical consciousness-raising of health and social care inequalities, identified from lobbying and evidence-based practice (research) |

**Figure 6.2**  The empowerment model

- *Evidence-based practice* was identified as part of the National Service Frameworks and assisted in referring Brian to experts who could help him improve his mobility and manage his diabetes.
- *Environmental issues* were identified in that Brian lives in a very rural area, making transport for shopping and hospital appointments difficult.
- Brian's *physical needs* were identified as being important to help him maintain some independence and develop other areas of his life now that he has retired.
- Brian's *psychological needs* required him to make some adjustments to how he felt about his health and lifestyle and what he could do to feel more positive.
- Brian's *social needs* were also dependent on his ability to get to places, meet people and socialize. Once his physical needs were more under control he could concentrate on improving his quality of life.
- Brian had in the past addressed his *spiritual needs* through religion but is now happy just keeping in contact with his brother and a few friends. He is now developing new skills in art as a new hobby.

The quality agenda and the empowerment model are useful tools in auditing the actions taken to help individuals progress towards more independent living. Practitioners are not always aware of how important the auditing process is in demonstrating that they are in fact providing good quality care. Everyone needs feedback including staff, clients, carers and even managers. Good quality care planning becomes very evident in the way we obtain, document and provide information for each and every person we work with.

**Practice point: the auditing process**

In your own area of practice, audits may be taking place all the time regarding the care planning process. You may not be aware that they are even happening. Next time you meet with your manager ask them about case note audits and if there is a checklist available in your workplace. This will enable you to check your own performance all the time rather than waiting (often anxiously) for the results of an audit.

## Chapter summary

➡ The quality agenda helps us to evaluate service provision and improve the care planning process.
➡ Practitioners must take into account the client's narrative of their experience of the process or journey.
➡ Changes can be made to improve practice based upon experience and understanding of the care planning process.
➡ Keeping the client centre stage in the whole process will help us to avoid alienation and poor quality practice.

## Self-assessment questions

What are the main areas of the quality agenda?

How can we keep the client at the centre of the care planning process?

What can you use to check that you have covered all the areas of the care planning process?

How can you check that you have the knowledge and skills to carry out your part in the care planning process?

# 7 Care planning policy in the UK

## This chapter will help you to:

➡ Outline the policy that drives current health and social care.
➡ Identify political influences on health and social care planning.
➡ Discuss clinical and social governance frameworks.
➡ Outline the different roles and responsibilities of particular health and social care providers.

## Introduction

*The prospects and possibilities of policy over the next few years will clearly be affected by the kind of society and culture that has taken shape, and the kind of context it provides for policy development.*

(Malin *et al.* 2002: 4)

In this chapter we will explore in some detail the management and organization of care from a wider perspective in order to reflect upon how this influences care planning in everyday practice. The health and social care system in the UK has become a multidisciplinary practice which has developed over time as a result of frequent restructuring and reorganization towards a more market-led, consumer-oriented approach (Malin *et al.* 2002). While it has many benefits, the multidisciplinary approach can lead to people no longer being sure where to obtain the health and social care services they need. An understanding of the process of planning health and social care provision is therefore necessary if we are to act as guides to people in need of care (Green 2007). This chapter aims to provide a simplistic overview of the system and the different sectors that provide health and social care. These sectors are also sometimes known as 'stakeholders'. We will briefly look at the quality agenda in health and social care and how this is planned and managed – in particular the need to recognize why the quality agenda has become increasingly important for all those who deliver health and social care.

## Political influences on current health and social care

In 1997, the government attempted to change the way health care was delivered in the NHS by introducing clinical governance and the 'third way' for publicly funded resources. Malin *et al.* (2002) suggest that the third way was an attempt to join methods of working together to develop a more collaborative approach to delivering health and social care services. The term 'devolution' is now common in many areas where political decision-making takes place and in the health care arena there has been a deliberate attempt to shift responsibility for health and social care nearer to home; for example, commissioning voluntary and private organizations to provide services that were once provided by the NHS. In the policy document *The New NHS: Modern, Dependable* (DoH 1997) three very important changes to health care delivery were proposed:

- The removal of Crown immunity against prosecution for failure to meet the needs of the public. The policy suggested that all NHS trusts should become responsible for their own actions, with the result that all trusts were required to assess and become aware of risk.
- All practice should be evidence based with the best available evidence being used to support practice interventions. The resources of the NHS were being stretched beyond capacity at that time and so it was deemed reasonable to expect that those resources should be targeted towards practice that was proven to be effective. NICE was set up to identify the best available evidence and produce guidance for consumers and practitioners within the NHS.
- The establishment of a monitoring system that would audit NHS trusts and communicate with patients to establish whether their care was based on the best available evidence and had been adapted to meet their individual needs. The Commission for Health Improvement (CHI) was created to do this and was later renamed the Healthcare Commission. The name was changed yet again in 2009 to the Care Quality Commission (CQC) to reflect the wider quality agenda of health and social care.

Social care delivery was also targeted in the reorganization of the NHS in 1997 with funding for local services being devolved to local authorities, primary care trusts (PCTs) and/or local health boards. These commissioning groups consist of cross-disciplinary members, including health and social care providers, delivering services in response to local need.

Social care involves a range of professionals who are employed by local authorities to address local, individual and group needs. Social workers are registered professionals who are qualified and registered with the General Social Care Council (GSCC) to act as caseworkers and advocates, assessing risk and promoting empowerment and social change (DoH 2006a).

---

**Hot topic**

Is health and social care too bureaucratic? How could we make access to services easier? This chapter will help you to reflect on some of the political and bureaucratic influences on your day-to-day practice.

---

## The role of the World Health Organization

Targets now drive many health and social care providers, reflecting any reduction of particular identified local needs through health and social care promotion, or any increase in health and social care activities that are likely to improve health and well-being. The World Health Organization (WHO 1998) continues to develop strategies based on evaluative research that will reduce inequalities in health and social care across Europe and the world, promoting health and reducing the burden of disease. The WHO's mission statement is that 'health is one of the fundamental rights of every human being. Health is a precondition for well-being and the quality of life. It is the benchmark for measuring progress towards the reduction of poverty, the promotion of social cohesion and the elimination of discrimination' (WHO 1998: 8).

Three ethical values form the basis of the WHO's strategy:

- health as a fundamental human right;
- equity in health and solidarity in action between and within all countries and their inhabitants; and
- participation and accountability.

The above values should therefore be found in every health and social care team across the UK and Europe in an effort to promote the health lifestyles of each and every individual person. Together with the changes in the UK NHS and social care system, providing good quality care is now the responsibility of every person involved through participation in care planning decisions and being accountable for decisions taken.

## Quality in health and social care

Everyone who is in receipt of health and social care and who works in such environments should be concerned with the quality management of the service. The NHS *Knowledge and Skills Framework* (DoH 2004) defines this as a core dimension (Dimension 5) of practice and suggests that staff at all levels should incorporate quality measures into their own work in order to help their service develop. The document suggests that quality improvement can occur in a number of ways, including:

- *team working:* demonstrating a commitment to your work and your colleagues in identifying issues and helping to find solutions;

- *role fulfilment:* making sure that you fulfil your role (or job description), fully understand the role of others in the NHS and respect their different approaches to practice;
- *policy development:* contributing to and carrying out local and national policy, including legal and ethical guidance and professional codes of conduct.

Using quality as a focus helps us to see where services might be improved or are working well in addressing local needs. Poor quality care will inevitably cost the organization, whether in terms of legal costs or repairs to worn out resources. One of the biggest areas of good quality health and social care provision is in training staff to carry out their work efficiently and effectively, as no matter how much money is provided to the service, if practitioners do not know how to deliver good quality care then the core objectives of the service will not be met (SCIE 2007).

---

**Practice point**

It is important to bear in mind when reading documents such as the *Knowledge and Skills Framework* (DoH 2004) that team working is an essential part of any quality improvement process and that while each individual can make changes to their practice it is ultimately the whole team or system that has the greater effect. This can be very frustrating for individual dynamic members of staff who are more than willing to play their part in improving services but find that without the whole team being on board with new initiatives, they are often destined to fail. This can lead to staff burnout where people stop trying to make changes to their practice because it feels too much like an uphill struggle. They will eventually give up if not supported by their managers and colleagues. Team working is discussed in more detail in Chapters 3 and 5.

---

Clinical and social care planning or 'governance' (DoH 1997, 2002a) does not just apply to professional staff but to everyone working in the NHS and social care.

Quality in health and social care has been identified as the only way to provide an efficient and effective service that can lead to the recovery and independence of people and groups in the community. The quality assurance framework bears a close similarity to individual and local care planning that aims to target resources where they are needed most (SCIE 2007). Local authorities and planning boards are therefore requested on a regular basis to provide a plan of how resources will be delivered in the local area. However, these decisions are also influenced by government and their inspections of clinical and social governance, or by the results of a serious inquiry (DoH 2000a). For example, following the report on the tragic case of Victoria Climbié, who died following extended abuse and neglect from her carers, all local authorities have been required to have plans in place for recording children's needs if they are at risk and for communicating those plans quickly and coherently (DoH 2003a: 34):

*Each local authority with social services responsibilities must establish a Committee of Members for Children and Families with lay members drawn from the management committees of each of the key services. This Committee must ensure the services to children and families are properly coordinated and that the inter-agency dimension of this work is being managed effectively.*

However, recommendations alone do not secure services and the above case has been found to be repeated too many times since the report by Lord Laming in 2003. It is because of tragic cases such as these that services must decide how their resources are used wisely and with great attention being paid to individual as well as local needs.

---

**Activity 7.1**

Read the following news article and consider how the issues raised might affect the quality of health and social care.

Watchdog tells doctors to prescribe fewer antibiotics

*Doctors have been told to stop routinely giving out antibiotics for common coughs, in an attempt to save the NHS millions of pounds. The over-prescription of antibiotics has been linked to the rise of drug-resistant superbugs. Around 38 million prescriptions for antibiotics were written by GPs in the UK last year, costing the NHS £175 million. NICE advises doctors to tell patients suffering from respiratory infections that they do not need antibiotics, or to offer them a delayed prescription. Patients should be reassured that antibiotics will 'make little difference to symptoms and may have side-effects', it states.*

(*The Guardian*, 23 July 2008)

---

## Factors when considering local needs

The following factors must be considered by all health and social care planning teams and should also be based on the best available evidence such as NICE guidelines.

- *Individual needs* – how many people in the locality need a particular service identified from their individual assessments? For example, if only one person suffers from one illness (which would probably be a rare illness of some sort), it would be unlikely that a service for that illness would be provided locally and they would have to travel further afield to access help.
- *Local needs* – of specific health and social care groups, for example, if a large proportion of a population are elderly, which is often the case in areas of the county where people move to retire. If there was a huge demand for a certain type of service then it would probably be cost effective to provide it locally rather than refer it to other service providers. However, some voluntary organizations now

provide services locally on commission from the local authority or through individual fundraising events. Unfortunately, these services are not always reliable because, due to the complex nature of bidding to obtain funds, many local organizations continue to rely heavily on fundraising events and are unable to plan services in the long term.

- *Accessibility* – whether the service is available nearby or is provided by another organization and can be 'bought in'. Sometimes this will lead to a competitive market for certain services and therefore should always be monitored by the funding body, which is usually the health and/or local authority.
- *Resources* – each local area will develop their resources as required in response to local need. However, these resources will also need to be constantly reviewed in terms of their being an effective way to deliver services. A good example would be the closure of some local day services when they are no longer being used or if that service can be provided more efficiently elsewhere.

---

### Activity 7.2

Often students on health and social care courses are asked to go and find out about the services available in their own locality. This is not a wasted exercise and if you have not already been asked to do this it is strongly recommended that you do so as soon as possible. Making a list of local organizations, contact numbers and names, which can be kept in an accessible place, can save everyone a great deal of time when creating individual care plans and can make the transition from hospital to home or vice versa a great deal less stressful for patients.

---

## Strategic management of resources

In relation to the clinical and social governance agenda, when considering the strategic management and allocation of resources, managers are usually expected to put forward a plan of care based on the needs of the population. They will also be requested to provide regular reports or audits of how their resources have been managed and what training needs have been identified and provided. Managers will also be expected to include the evidence for why resources are being organized in a certain way and how they have involved clients in gathering that evidence. Finally, managers and their organizations will need to demonstrate how they have managed any risks to individuals and the organizations themselves. While many of you reading this book will feel far removed from the strategic level of service organization and delivery as part of the clinical and social governance framework, we are all responsible for our actions. As a consequence of following the activities in this book you may now be more aware of the many different people and policies involved in a single person's care that will need to be considered in your own area of practice. This is not always something that as practitioners we are informed about during our practice, but we nevertheless tend to find out about as we go along. Managers of staff will have a greater awareness of the clinical and social governance frameworks, but awareness by all staff will make the process much quicker and smoother. There may well be areas of the framework that you cannot access, but an acknowledgment of what might be available will help you to help patients like Brian or advocate on their behalf to access good quality care. However, just as the framework for good quality care is important, so is a basic understanding of the structure of health and social care provision and this will be explored in more depth below.

# Overview of the structure and management of health and social care in the UK

When planning care it is necessary to bear in mind the series of stages that planning and organization go through that can lead to delays in, or a complete lack of, services in some areas, as explained above. Services and organizations may appear to work in complete isolation but in reality they are all reliant upon one another. The main organizations are outlined below and are not meant to represent a hierarchical structure of power but a picture of the various stages an idea that is first identified in one place as being an improvement will go through, taking a variety of routes to reach its intended recipient. It is hardly surprising that by the time it reaches the recipient it may have been diluted to a considerable extent. Ideas for changes in practice can come from the bottom up through client and carer involvement initiatives as well as from the top down. In fact, most policy or reporting documents now include stories or narratives of clients and their carers. In other countries some of the layers may not exist and so the roles and responsibilities of each department that does exist will be commensurately greater.

---

**Practice point: who does what in the quality agenda?**

In practice it can become very confusing regarding who does what and where within the quality agenda. This chapter is designed to help you see how many different organizations may be involved in just one person's care.

---

The hierarchy of care

Parliament or the governing body for each country within the UK is where major decisions are made about health and social care. Social policy and sometimes law is produced by the government to guide local and regional departments in how their budgets should be spent and practice developed. This may be based on research evidence for certain treatments or services and/or in order to promote health and independence. The guidelines developed by the government in question may be monitored by other agencies commissioned by that government such as the national quality inspection bodies identified above. Since the late 1990s the UK government has targeted health and social care as an area of improvement and decided to give more responsibility to local areas for planning their services. This is known as clinical and/or social governance, and local services are expected to improve standards of care as a result. One of the fundamental documents to come out of this restructuring in England was the *Essence of Care* patient-focused benchmarks in 2001 (DoH 2003c). Consequent inspections of health and social care organizations are often based on these benchmarks for which further guidance has been developed that includes communication, promoting health and the care environment.

## Strategic and regional health and local authorities

These authorities are responsible for deciding how services should be developed in their area. This is important because the government is aware that some areas of the country may need different services to others. For instance, rural areas will need services that can be accessed more locally. Strategic and regional health authorities will still need to follow the above benchmarks but may adapt resources to meet some of their own area's need.

Local authorities, like regional health authorities, are responsible for deciding how services that are not provided by health authorities are delivered in the local area. This will include health-promoting activities on a wider scale (e.g. public health initiatives such as health education and sanitation as well as direct support for social services departments).

## Primary health care teams/local health boards/health and social care departments

These teams are funded by the strategic and/or regional health authorities and have an influence on how health care resources will be dispersed in primary care in each county. They are accountable to the strategic and/or regional authorities and must provide justification for how they decide resources should be used. They are composed of a multidisciplinary team/board and therefore should be able to agree on health care provision using a whole-care or whole-systems approach. This means that they have considered all the health care needs of a group of individuals and not just one aspect (e.g. medication).

## Social services departments

Social services departments are based within local authorities and provide or commission health and social care across the lifespan from the very young to the very old. Social services therefore have to manage a wide diversity of needs and often work very closely with the voluntary and private sectors. Social services departments also have a wider involvement in the local community and in identifying and addressing the needs of that local community.

## Primary health care

Primary care is known as such because it is usually the first point of contact for an individual or group requiring health care. This generally means the GP surgery where a patient will be assessed by the doctor and/or nurse and either provided with care or referred on to secondary care or other services. This is usually required when a specialist service is needed, as in the case of, for example, heart disease, although a large majority of people living in the community are wholly taken care of in primary care. The primary care team will provide health promotion, health education and the monitoring of health care for people with mild to moderate needs. Primary care services are responsible for the budget for prescription medications and for helping their patients choose and plan appropriate health care from secondary services. Primary care also includes walk-in centres, dentistry, opticians and NHS Direct.

## Secondary health care

Secondary care can only be accessed directly through accident and emergency departments. All other routes into secondary care must be through the primary care team. Secondary care provides more specialist interventions and treatments for disorders such as heart disease, cancer, mental illness and diabetes. There are many other disorders that are treatable within the secondary care services but they must all follow the basic care standards set out in the *Essence of Care* document identified above.

## Voluntary and private sector care

The voluntary and private sectors are a growing and rapidly developing contribution to health and social care provision. Developed largely from the market-driven and consumer movements, services are organized around those areas that are perhaps not already provided within the statutory provision. For example, some organizations provide private care to people who suffer from alcohol and drug addictions. Similarly, different charity groups such as Mind or Help the Aged provide support and befriending services. These charitable agencies are also known as 'third sector organizations' (TSOs) and are supported by the government to plan and provide alternative resources and a voice for certain sectors of the community who may be hard to reach (National Audit Office 2005).

# Partnership working

---

**Activity 7.3**

Brian had a number of needs that were identified in his care plan. Take a brief look at the above organizations and consider which of them were involved in Brian's care. See below for the answers.

---

Health and social care planning spans a variety of organizations, who are all guided by local and national policy. Social policy has therefore become a major influence in everyday practice and clinical and social governance plays a large part in ensuring that social policy in the form of laws and guidelines is implemented. Each organization is responsible for the planning or governance of its own resources and for providing evidence of how that has been carried out. It has become essential that organizations communicate with each other about their local needs and plans (Carnwell and Buchanan 2005). In addition, whenever things have gone tragically wrong in health and social care the problem can usually be found to have developed from a communication breakdown within or between services. The importance of working in partnership with other agencies is frequently recommended in government reports and is often a requirement when bidding for funding or extra resources. However, this could be seen as a threat to many professional organizations that prefer to continue in their usual practice and routines, but it is becoming increasingly difficult *not* to work in partnership with other agencies.

In relation to Activity 7.3, which asked you to identify which organizations were involved in Brian's care, the following might be a typical scenario:

- *Primary care* services were involved because Brian is registered with a GP who is responsible for his overall care needs and was also working in partnership with the practice nurse and the pharmacist in making sure Brian had regular blood tests and his insulin was available.
- *Secondary care* services were involved because Brian needed help from a diabetic specialist nurse and/or doctor. Brian agreed to attend a regular diabetic clinic in the local hospital where they could help him use the best available evidence in managing his diabetes. The clinic staff also needed to keep his GP informed of any changes made to Brian's medication and/or diet.
- *Voluntary care* services were available in the form of a support group or befriending service which helped Brian manage his diabetes based on other people's experiences with the same condition.
- *Social services* were involved with Brian to help him organize transport and other activities.

## Planning care across organizations

Care planning features as a large part of the services that are delivered by the above organizations. While it is important for local areas and services to plan for the provision of care of a whole group of people, at this level services are not so concerned with individual care planning. Service organizations do however need to come together to manage the overall care, planned in the most efficient and effective way possible and in line with the clinical and social governance agenda. The DoH is looking at how this can be achieved by providing guidance – in supporting people with long-term conditions, for example (DoH 2005). The DoH suggests the need for a systematic approach towards planning health and social care that corresponds to the level of complexity and dependency of groups and/or individuals. The important message is that we must not treat all people with health and social care needs as being the same. While there may be a number of people like Brian, for example, who suffer from a long-term condition, they may not all have the same level of need. It is up to the organizations concerned to put in place systems and policies that are flexible enough to help them decide how best to meet local needs. The levels of organization are not therefore a hierarchy of eligibility that only the people with the most needs will qualify for, but a suggested system for care planning across organizations that will be of the most benefit to different clients.

## National Service Frameworks and minimum standards

When the government identified that health and social care needed to be more quality-focused it developed standards that were measurable for services provided to particular patient groups. These groups are people who suffer from a condition that depends greatly upon health and social care services. They include people who suffer from long-term conditions and other major diseases such as heart disease, mental health problems, cancer and diabetes. Minimum standards are used to assess the quality of care in registered services such as home care, care agencies and voluntary and residential services.

## The Health and Social Care Act 2008

In July 2008 royal approval was given for a new law on governing health and social care which would abolish the Healthcare Commission, the Mental Health Act Commission and the Commission for Social Care Inspection and replace them with a new overarching quality monitoring system. This is known as the Care Quality Commission (CQC) and oversees three main areas of quality inspection:

- the improvement of health and social care services including health and safety, infection control, risk assessment, professional regulation, education and training etc.;
- the monitoring of the efficacy and effectiveness of health and social care services and the implementation of evidence-based practice;
- the inclusion of clients and carers in decisions about their care and the provision of direct payments for them to become more empowered in addressing their individual needs.

---

**Hot topic**

When *guidelines* are made into *law* it is possible to be prosecuted if such a law is broken (guidelines tend to be more flexible). In your own area of practice (and perhaps during supervision) you may want to spend some time with your supervisor/mentor to consider the three main areas of the Health and Social Care Act 2008 and identify aspects of risk/practice that may bring prosecutions in the future.

---

## Planning for care at the local level and in teams

This is the point where managers have to designate and allocate all the resources that have been assigned at the prior planning levels described above to meet the health care needs of their own local population. There have been various reorganizations of the administrative and management structures at a local level in recent years, and there are probably more ahead, so some general principles of line management for practitioners working in health and social care will be used here. Readers and care practitioners should make themselves aware of the personnel and management structure at this level and for any area in which they are working.

---

**Activity 7.4**

Discuss with your mentor or manager the levels of management within your own organization. Find out the roles and responsibilities of each person and create a chart for your portfolio demonstrating how they might influence your day-to-day work.

---

Whatever team you belong to, from time to time you and your colleagues will need to look at how you prioritize and organize care. Depending on the environment in which you work, this may take place at regular, structured team meetings, perhaps on a weekly basis, such as referral meetings, caseload meetings or alternatively daily ward handovers. These meetings are usually led by a senior member of the team who is accountable for good quality care provision. Senior members of the team will be expected to have knowledge of and be able to consider all the health and social governance areas identified above, and will be making day-to-day decisions on how best they can be met and adhered to. So while you may only be thinking of what you need to be doing that day, the great cogs of a huge organization are constantly turning. Senior staff members will then be expected to feed back to *their* managers with regard to any concerns the team may have about providing good quality care. It is therefore *your responsibility* to make it known to your managers any concerns that you have about your own competence and the resources available to carry out your work. Even though you may not be professionally accountable at this stage in your development you can be accountable to your educational establishment under suitability to practice policies and/or the law if your actions have led to the harm of a vulnerable person or group (NMC 2005).

Often senior managers are required to provide evidence of regular caseload/case note audits and this usually requires an examination of a group of people's care records to see if every part of their individual care plans is complete. This is where documentation becomes very important as in most professional organizations, as we have emphasized throughout this book, the general rule is that *if it has not been documented it has not been done*. The Mental Capacity Act 2005 has addressed this issue in suggesting that if it has not been documented as to *why* it has not been done then it may also be deemed as neglectful practice.

Whatever level of care planning you are personally involved in it is important therefore to recognize and understand how the whole process works and what you and the client can expect from health and social care services. With a basic understanding of the organizations, laws, knowledge and skills required to support such a large system we can all contribute to a better quality service.

---

## Chapter summary

➡ Clinical and social governance was introduced to improve the quality of health and social care.

➡ There are many organizations that provide services, directed by government.

➡ Local services must plan and organize care that is responsive to local need.

➡ Partnership working across organizations will improve the efficiency and effectiveness of the care delivered.

➡ Documentation and audit are the main ways in which good quality care can be evidenced and the opportunity for improvements identified.

---

## Self-assessment questions

What is the role and philosophy of the service that you provide?

How will case note audit help you to identify good quality practice?

What levels of line management are there in your organization?

What are the three main areas of quality inspection under the Health and Social Care Act 2008?

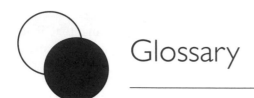

# Glossary

| Term | Definition |
|---|---|
| **Care coordinator** | The person who organizes health and/or social care. They may also be called the 'key worker' or the 'primary care worker', depending on the area of practice. The care coordinator can also be the person's GP if they are the only person involved in providing care. |
| **Care pathway** | A care pathway is a previously designed care plan focused on a particular disease or type of service provision. Care pathways offer an outline of a standard of care that can be expected by an individual. |
| **Care plan** | A written, typed or electronic document that states what care will be provided for a client, signed by the care coordinator and the client. It should clearly state the person's needs, goals and the relevant interventions, and include a review (evaluation) date for each need/goal (some organizations use separate care plans for each type of need). |
| **Carer** | A person who provides *unpaid* care for another person. They may be an adult, older person or child. |
| **Client** | A person receiving care who may also be known as a 'patient' or 'consumer', depending on the area of practice. |
| **Clinical and social governance** | The way in which care is organized and provided to ensure quality. This applies to organizational and individual care provision and should be transparent in all that we do. |
| **Continuing professional development (CPD)** | Employers are expected to make sure that practitioners/employees are able to develop their skills where necessary to improve their practice and the quality of care provided. Training and educational needs in any organization should therefore be based on CPD and clinical/social governance outcomes (and not individual preferences, as is sometimes the case). This is a health and safety issue as much as a personal development one, but the two need to be addressed together to improve care. |

| National Health Service (NHS) | Includes all areas that provide health care including different professional groups and private and voluntary organizations, the funding for which primarily comes from the same budget. Many policy documents that refer to the NHS are also relevant to private and voluntary health care sectors. |
|---|---|
| Practitioner | Any person who is working with a client. They may or may not be the care coordinator and may or may not be registered with a professional body. They are, however, *paid* workers from the health, social care or voluntary sector. |
| Reflection | A process of reviewing practice or an event based on a particular theory or evidence base that will lead to a changed outcome. |
| Risk | The chance that something harmful will happen. Positive risk is when this is acknowledged as being at an acceptable level, but risk can change and hence needs constant observation and monitoring. |
| Social care | The provision of support in helping people maintain or improve their place in the community. This may involve people working in housing, education, welfare, occupational or recreational settings. |
| Stakeholder | Any person who is involved in providing and/or receiving care. |
| Supervision | A regular meeting between two people or a group of people where reflection on practice takes place concerning an individual client. The supervisor may also be known as your 'mentor', 'practice teacher' or 'preceptor'. (*Caseload supervision* is different in that it is usually carried out with a manager and is organizational rather than practice-focused.) |

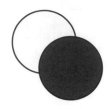

# Recommended reading

Blakemore, K. and Griggs, E. (2007) *Social Policy: An Introduction*. Buckingham: Open University Press.

Bradshaw, P.L. and Bradshaw, G. (2004) *Health Policy for Health Care Professionals*. London: Sage.

Brotherton, G. and Parker, S. (2007) *Your Foundation in Health and Social Care: A Guide for Foundation Degree Students*. London: Sage.

Fraser, S. and Matthews, S. (2007) *The Critical Practitioner in Social Work and Health Care*. London: Sage.

Hargie, O. (2006) *The Handbook of Communication Skills*, 3rd edn. London: Routledge.

Hek, G. and Moule, P. (2006) *Making Sense of Research: An Introduction for Health and Social Care Practitioners*, 3rd edn. London: Sage.

Iles, V. (2006) *Really Managing Health Care*, 2nd edn. Maidenhead: Open University Press.

Johnson, J. and De Souza, C. (2008) *Understanding Health and Social Care: An Introductory Reader*. London: Sage.

Leathard, A. (2003) *Interprofessional Collaboration: From Policy to Practice in Health and Social Care*. New York: Brunner Routledge.

Lloyd, M. and Murphy, P. (2008) *Essential Study Skills in Health and Social Care*. Exeter: Reflect Press.

MacSherry, R. and Warr, J. (2008) *An Introduction to Excellence in Practice Development in Health and Social Care*. Maidenhead: Open University Press.

Malone, C., Forbat, L., Robb, M. and Seden, J. (2005) *Relating Experience: Stories from Health and Social Care*. London: Routledge.

Martin, V. and Henderson, E. (2010) *Managing in Health and Social Care*, 2nd edn. London: Routledge.

Peckham, S. and Meerabeau, B. (2007) *Social Policy for Nurses and the Helping Professions*. Maidenhead: Open University Press.

Penhale, B. and Parker, J. (2008) *Working with Vulnerable Adults*. London: Routledge.

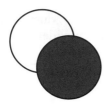

# Websites for further information and advice

| Organization | Web address | What they do |
| --- | --- | --- |
| **British Association/ College of Occupational Therapists** | www.cot.co.uk | A professional body that provides information free to the public including a professional code of ethics |
| **British Association of Social Workers** | www.basw.co.uk | A professional group where members can identify with a code of ethics and discuss practice issues |
| **Care Quality Commission** | www.cqc.org.uk | A new organization that replaces the Healthcare Commission, Mental Health Act Commission and the Social Care Inspectorate in England |
| **Care Services Improvement Programme (CSIP)** | www.csip.org.uk | Promotes good quality social care through policy development and implementation |
| **Department of Health (DoH)** | www.dh.gov.uk | Provides access to many policy documents which can be downloaded or ordered from the website |
| **Diabetes UK** | www.diabetes.org.uk | Provides information on self-management of diabetes |
| **DIPEX** | www.dipex.org | Provides personal stories on a wide variety of health and illness and how services contribute to care provision |

| General Social Care Council (GSCC) | www.gscc.org.uk | Provides and monitors codes of conduct for all social care workers and provides professional advice |
|---|---|---|
| Health and Safety Executive (HSE) | www.hse.gov.uk | A very useful website with lots of free information on managing risk in the workplace |
| INVOLVE | www.invo.org.uk | A public advisory group that provides guidance on involving clients in research |
| National Institute for Health and Clinical Excellence (NICE) | www.nice.org.uk | Provides evidence-based practice for a range of conditions and treatments |
| National Institute for Mental Health (England) (NIMHE) | www.nimhe.csip.org.uk | A division of CSIP that focuses on improving services for people with mental health problems |
| NHS Library | www.library.nhs.uk | Provides information on a variety of illnesses |
| Nursing and Midwifery Council (NMC) | www.nmc-uk.org | Provides code of conduct and professional advice and regulation for nurses and midwives |
| Office of the Public Guardian (OPG) | www.publicguardian.gov.uk | Provides information on helping a person make decisions if they risk losing capacity at any time |
| Royal College of Nursing (RCN) | www.rcn.org.uk | A professional group that provides support and advice for nurses and health care workers |
| Skills for Care | www.skillsforcare.org.uk | Aims to improve standards of care in social care through education, practice and competency development (e.g. National Occupational Standards) |

| Skills for Health | www.skillsfor-health.org.uk | Aims to improve standards of care in health care through education, practice and competency development (e.g. Knowledge and Skills Framework) |
|---|---|---|
| Social Care Institute for Excellence (SCIE) | www.scie.org.uk | Provides evidence of good practice within health and social care |
| Unison | www.unison.org.uk | A trade union for all health and social care staff. This organization offers publications and guidance to people who are non-members as well as members |

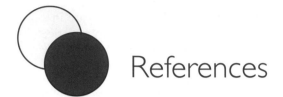

# References

Allison, A. (2005) The ethical issues of working in partnership, in R. Carnwell and J. Buchanan (eds) *Effective Practice in Health and Social Care: A Partnership Approach*. Maidenhead: Open University Press.

Berreta, R. (2003) Assessment: foundation of good practice, in S. Hinchcliff, A. Norman and J Schober (eds) *Nursing Practice and Health Care*. London: Arnold.

Brindle, D. (2008) Baby P case raises questions over child protection practice, *Society Guardian* (11 November).

British Association of Social Workers (2002) *The Code of Ethics for Social Work*. Birmingham: BASW, available to download at www.basw.co.uk/Default.aspx?tabid=64.

Carnwell, R. and Buchanan, J. (2005) *Effective Practice in Health and Social Care: A Partnership Approach*. Maidenhead: Open University Press.

Church, K. (1995) *Forbidden Narratives: Critical Autobiography as Social Science*. London: Routledge.

College for Occupational Therapists (2005) *Code of Ethics and Professional Conduct*, available at www.cot.org.uk.

DoH (Department of Health) (1997) *The New NHS: Modern, Dependable*. London: HMSO, available at www.dh.gov.uk/en/Publicationsandstatistics/Publications/PublicationsPolicyAndGuidance/DH_4008869.

DoH (Department of Health) (2000a) *An Organisation with a Memory: Report from an Expert Group on Learning from Adverse Events*. London: HMSO, available at www.dh.gov.uk/en/Publicationsandstatistics/Lettersandcirculars/Dearcolleagueletters/DH_4005264.

DoH (Department of Health) (2000b) *No Secrets: Guidance on Developing and Implementing Multiagency Policies and Procedures to Protect Vulnerable Adults from Abuse*. London: HMSO, available at www.dh.gov.uk/en/Publicationsandstatistics/Publications/PublicationsPolicyAndGuidance/DH_4008486.

DoH (Department of Health) (2001a) *National Service Framework for Diabetes: Standards*. London: HMSO, available at www.dh.gov.uk/en/Publicationsandstatistics/Publications/PublicationsPolicyAndGuidance/DH_4002951.

DoH (Department of Health) (2001b) *The Expert Patient: A New Approach to Chronic Disease Management in the 21st Century*. London: HMSO, available at

www.dh.gov.uk/en/Publicationsandstatistics/Publications/
PublicationsPolicyAndGuidance/DH_4006801.

DoH (Department of Health) (2001c) *National Service Framework for Older People.* London: HMSO.

DoH (Department of Health) (2002a) *Quality in Social Care: The National Institutional Framework.* London: HMSO, available at www.dh.gov.uk/en/
Publicationsandstatistics/Publications/PublicationsPolicyAndGuidance/DH_4084025.

DoH (Department of Health) (2002b) *The Single Assessment Process: Single Assessment Summary – Worked Example.* London: HMSO, available at www.dh.gov.uk/en/
Publicationsandstatistics/Publications/PublicationsPolicyAndGuidance/DH_4009402.

DoH (Department of Health) (2003a) *The Victoria Climbié Inquiry. Report of an Inquiry by Lord Laming.* London: HMSO, available at www.dh.gov.uk/en/
Publicationsandstatistics/Lettersandcirculars/Dearcolleagueletters/DH_4008676.

DoH (Department of Health) (2003b) *Fair Access to Care Services: Guidance on Eligibility Criteria for Adult Social Care.* London: HMSO, available at www.dh.gov.uk/
en/Publicationsandstatistics/Publications/PublicationsPolicyAndGuidance/
DH_4009653.

DoH (Department of Health) (2003c) *Essence of Care: Patient Focused Benchmarks for Clinical Governance.* London: NHS Modernization Agency, available at
www.dh.gov.uk/en/Publicationsandstatistics/Publications/
PublicationsPolicyAndGuidance/DH_4005475.

DoH (Department of Health) (2003d) *Discharge from Hospital Pathway: Process and Practice.* London: HMSO, available at www.dh.gov.uk/en/Publicationsandstatistics/
Publications/PublicationsPolicyAndGuidance/DH_4003252.

DoH (Department of Health) (2004) *The Knowledge and Skills Framework and the Developmental Review Process.* London: HMSO, available at www.dh.gov.uk/en/
Publicationsandstatistics/Publications/PublicationsPolicyAndGuidance/DH_4090843.

DoH (Department of Health) (2005a) *Supporting People with Long Term Conditions: An NHS and Social Care Model to Support Local Innovation and Integration.* London: HMSO, available at www.dh.gov.uk/en/Publicationsandstatistics/Publications/
PublicationsPolicyAndGuidance/DH_4100252.

DoH (Department of Health) (2005b) *National Service Framework for Long Term Conditions.* London: HMSO, available at www.dh.gov.uk/en/
Publicationsandstatistics/Publications/PublicationsPolicyAndGuidance/DH_4105361.

DoH (Department of Health) (2006a) *Our Health, Our Care, Our Say: A New Direction for Community Services.* London: HMSO, available at www.dh.gov.uk/en/
Publicationsandstatistics/Publications/PublicationsPolicyAndGuidance/Browsable/
DH_4127552.

DoH (Department of Health) (2006b) *Direct Payments for People with Mental Health Problems: A Guide to Action.* London: HMSO, available at www.dh.gov.uk/en/
Publicationsandstatistics/Publications/PublicationsPolicyAndGuidance/DH_4131060.

DoH (Department of Health) (2007a) *Independence, Choice and Risk: A Guide to Best Practice in Decision-making* (Appendix 1). London: HMSO, available at www.dh.gov.uk/en/Publicationsandstatistics/Publications/PublicationsPolicyAndGuidance/DH_074773.

DoH (Department of Health) (2007b) *Health Select Committee Inquiry into Patient and Public Involvement in the NHS*. London: HMSO, available at www.publications.parliament.uk/pa/cm200607/cmselect/cmhealth/278/278i.pdf.

DoH (Department of Health) (2008a) *Refocusing the Care Programme Approach: Policy and Positive Practice Guidance*. London: HMSO, available at www.dh.gov.uk/en/Publicationsandstatistics/Publications/PublicationsPolicyAndGuidance/DH_083647.

DoH (Department of Health) (2008b) *High Quality Care for All: NHS Next Stage Review Final Report*. London: HMSO, available at www.dh.gov.uk/en/Publicationsandstatistics/Publications/PublicationsPolicyAndGuidance/DH_085825.

Dziegielewski, S.F. (2004) *The Changing Face of Health Social Work: Professional Practice in Managed Behavioural Healthcare*, 2nd edn. New York: Springer.

Elliott, J. (2005) *Using Narrative in Social Research: Qualitative and Quantitative Approaches*. London: Sage.

Firth-Cozens, J. and Cornwell, J. (2009) *The Point of Care: Enabling Compassionate Care in Acute Hospital Settings*. London: The King's Fund.

Ghaye, T. (2000) The role of reflection in nurturing creative clinical conversations, in T. Ghaye and S. Lillyman (eds) *Effective Clinical Supervision: The Role of Reflection*. London: Quay Books.

Gibbs, G. (1988) *Learning by Doing: A Guide to Learning and Teaching Methods*. Oxford: Oxford Polytechnic.

Goffman, E. (1961) *Asylums: Essays on the Social Situation of Mental Patients and other Inmates*. Hammondsworth: Penguin.

Green, S. (2007) *Involving People in Healthcare Policy and Practice*. Oxford: Radcliffe.

Greenstreet, W. (2006) *Integrating Spirituality in Health and Social Care: Perspectives and Practical Approaches*. Oxford: Radcliffe.

Hawkins, P. and Shohet, R. (2006) *Supervision in the Helping Professions*, 3rd edn. Maidenhead: Open University Press.

Jaspers, M. (2003) *Beginning Reflective Practice*. Tewkesbury: Nelson Thornes.

Kitwood, T. (1997) *Dementia Reconsidered: The Person Comes First*. Buckingham: Open University Press.

Kleinman, A. (1988) *The Illness Narratives: Suffering Healing and the Human Condition*. New York: Basic Books.

Lindsay, B. (2007) *Understanding Research and Evidence-based Practice*. Exeter: Reflect Press.

Lloyd, M. (2007) Empowerment in the interpersonal field discourses of mental health nurses in the acute setting, *Journal of Psychiatric and Mental Health Nursing*, 14(5): 485–94.

Lloyd, M. (2009) Mental health nursing in a rehabilitation and recovery context, in V. Clarke and A. Walsh (eds) *Fundamentals of Mental Health Nursing*. Oxford: Oxford University Press.

Malin, N., Wilmot, S. and Manthorpe, J. (2002) *Key Debates in Health and Social Policy*. Buckingham: Open University Press.

McKenna, H. (1997) *Nursing Models and Theories*. London: Routledge.

Minhas, A. (2005) Dependent upon outside help: reflections from a client, in R. Carnwell and J. Buchanan (eds) *Effective Practice in Health and Social Care: A Partnership Approach*. Maidenhead: Open University Press.

National Audit Office (2005) *Working with the Third Sector*. London: HMSO, available at www.nao.org.uk/publications/0506/working_with_the_third_sector.aspx.

NMC (Nursing and Midwifery Council) (2005) *An NMC Guide for Readers of Nursing and Midwifery*. London: NMC.

NMC (Nursing and Midwifery Council) (2007) *Record-keeping*. London: NMC.

NMC (Nursing and Midwifery Council) (2008) *The Code: Standards of Conduct, Performance and Ethics for Nurses and Midwives*. London: NMC, available at www.nmc-uk.org/aDisplayDocument.aspx?documentID=3954.

NTA (National Treatment Agency) (2006) *Care Planning Practice Guide*. London: National Treatment Agency for Substance Misuse, available at www.nta.nhs.uk/publications/documents/nta_care_planning_practice_guide_2006_cpg1.pdf.

QAA (Quality Assurance Agency) (2006) *Statement of common purpose for subject benchmark statements for the health and social care professions*, available at www.qaa.ac.uk/academicinfrastructure/benchmark/health/StatementofCommonPurpose06.asp.

Rogers, C. (1967) *On Becoming a Person: A Therapist's View of Psychotherapy*. London: Constable.

Schön, D.A. (1983) *The Reflective Practitioner: How Professionals Think in Action*. London: Temple Smith.

SCIE (Social Care Institute for Excellence) (2007) *Social Care Governance: A Practice Workbook*, available at www.scie.org.uk/publications/misc/governance.asp.

Smith, A. (2004) New ways of working, in S. Chilton, K. Melling, D. Drew and A. Clarridge (eds) *Nursing in the Community: An Essential Guide to Practice*. London: Arnold.

Smith, M. (2004) Conceptual approaches to care, in S. Chilton, K. Melling, D. Drew and A. Clarridge (eds) *Nursing in the Community: An Essential Guide to Practice*. London: Arnold.

Stockwell, F. (1972) *The Unpopular Patient*. London: Royal College of Nursing, available at www.rcn.org.uk/__data/assets/pdf_file/0005/235508/series_1_number_2.pdf.

The Open University (1997) *A Systematic Approach to Nursing Care: An Exploration and Re-Evaluation*. Milton Keynes: The Open University.

Tones, K. (2001) Health promotion: the empowerment imperative, in A. Scriven and J. Orme (eds) *Health Promotion: Professional Perspectives*. Basingstoke: Palgrave.

Topss (2004) *The National Occupational Standards for Social Work*, available at www.york.ac.uk/depts/spsw/documents/3SWNOSdocpdffileseditionApr04.pdf.

Tummey, R. (2005) *Planning Care in Mental Health Nursing*. Basingstoke: Palgrave.

Unison (2003) *The Duty of Care: A Handbook to Assist Healthcare Staff to Carry out their Duty of Care to Patients, Colleagues and Themselves*. London: Unison, available at www.unison.org.uk/acrobat/13038.pdf.

Watson, D. and West, J. (2006) *Social Work Process and Practice: Approaches Knowledge and Skills*. Basingstoke: Palgrave Macmillan.

Watts, D. and Morgan, G. (1994) Malignant alienation: dangers for patients who are hard to like, *British Journal of Psychiatry*, 164: 11–15.

Welsh Assembly Government (2008) *Adult Mental Health Services, Stronger in Partnership 2: Involving Service Users and Carers in the Design, Planning, Delivery and Evaluation of Mental Health Services in Wales*. Cardiff: Welsh Assembly Government, available at www.wales.nhs.uk/documents/strongerpartner2e%5B1%5D.pdf.

WHO (World Health Organization) (1978) *Declaration of Alma-Ata*. Geneva: WHO.

WHO (World Health Organization) (1998) *Health 21: Health for all in the 21st Century*. Denmark: WHO, available at www.euro.who.int/document/ehfa5-e.pdf.

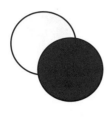

# Appendix: practice sheets and audit checklist

You can find printable downloads of all practice sheets online at:
www.openup.co.uk/careplanning

## Sheet 1: initial assessment

| **Completed by** .................................................... **Date** ....................... ||
|---|---|
| 1. Name of person being assessed | Address |
| Date of birth | Telephone number(s) |
| 2. Name of general practitioner | Address of general practitioner |
| | Telephone number of GP |
| 3. Name of next of kin | Address of next of kin |
| | Telephone number (s) |
| 4. Marital status<br>Married        Single<br>Divorced      Civil partnership<br>Other ................................... | 5. Religion |
| 6. Medication currently being taken (*add separate sheet if necessary*) | 7. Disabilities or impairments (*e.g. wears glasses, uses a hearing aid etc.*) |

| | |
|---|---|
| 8. Any known allergies? | 9. Dietary requirements |
| 10. Any dependants (*e.g. children, elderly parents etc.*)? | 11. Other agencies involved (*e.g. social worker, probation etc.*) |
| Contact details of dependants | Contact details of other agencies involved |
| 12. Current or previous occupation | 13. Any other requirements/urgent needs (*e.g. diabetes, epilepsy*) |

## Sheet 2: personal assessment

| Assessment information | Observations (please complete all boxes to show that they have been addressed) |
|---|---|
| **Biological: do you have any needs in the following areas?** | **Please state in the person's own words where possible and record any measurements (including frequency where required)** |
| Breathing | |
| Eating (including appetite) and food preparation | |
| Sleeping and rest | |
| Washing and bathing | |
| Dressing | |

| | |
|---|---|
| Moving and walking | |
| Exercise and activities | |
| Hygiene and self-care (*e.g. hair, nails, teeth, using the toilet, skin care etc.*) | |
| Maintaining/losing weight | |
| Vital signs: blood pressure, temperature, pulse, skin colour and texture | |
| **Psychological: do you have any needs in the following areas?** | |
| Memory | |
| Thought disturbances | |
| Moods and emotions | |
| Beliefs about others | |
| Perceptions | |
| Sensations (*e.g. taste, touch, smell, sight and sound*) | |

| Social: do you have any needs in the following areas? | |
| --- | --- |
| Family support | |
| Friends/peer support | |
| Meaningful occupation (*including work, hobbies etc.*) | |
| Group membership | |
| Recreational activities | |
| Significant relationships | |
| Spiritual: do you have any needs in the following areas? | |
| Personal religious beliefs | |
| Personal cultural beliefs | |

## Sheet 3: general risk assessment

| Area of risk | Current needs | Positive risks taken |
|---|---|---|
| Hypothermia | | |
| Neglect | | |
| Abuse, physical, emotional, financial | | |
| Exploitation | | |
| Slips, trips and falls | | |
| Isolation | | |
| Nutrition and hydration | | |
| Suicide/self-harm | | |
| Violence/aggression | | |

## Sheet 4: care plan using the SMART formula (*if only using one sheet remember to number needs in order of priority*)

| Patient name | | Date of birth | |
|---|---|---|---|
| **Needs** *(specific: in person's own words where possible)* | **Goals** *(Measurable and achievable: including any assessment tool measurements)* | **Interventions** *(Realistic)* | **Evaluation** *(Timely)* |
| | | | |

## Sheet 5: daily record sheet – to be completed by care coordinator or by designated person and countersigned by care coordinator

| Date | Record to be made at least once daily or on every contact | Signature and designa- tion |
|------|-----------------------------------------------------------|------------------------------|
|      |                                                           |                              |

## Checklist for care planning audit

| Evidence | Location in records (or noted for improvement and underlined) | Date and signature |
|---|---|---|
| Philosophy of care followed or professional codes/values adhered to | | |
| All paperwork signed and dated | | |
| Good record-keeping practices (e.g. factual, timely, non-judgemental, client involvement, jargon-free, SMART) | | |
| Initial assessment containing basic personal information and regularly updated | | |
| Full holistic assessment completed | | |
| Models and/or frameworks used | | |
| Risk assessment completed and updated at evaluation | | |
| Health and safety issues identified | | |
| Client's own words used | | |
| Client's needs identified | | |

| | | |
|---|---|---|
| Reflection upon practice | | |
| National Service Frameworks followed | | |
| Evidenced-based practice | | |
| Social policy/guidance followed | | |
| Application of relevant laws (e.g. Mental Capacity Act) | | |
| Personal and professional development identified | | |
| Team/multidisciplinary working | | |
| Resource allocation | | |
| Environmental and/or cultural needs identified | | |
| Other (specific to individual workplace) | | |

# Index

# ESSENTIAL CALCULATION SKILLS FOR NURSES AND MIDWIVES

**Meriel Hutton**

Calculation skills are a core part of nursing and midwifery practice, from calculating drug or medicine doses to monitoring a patients' liquid intake or stock management. It is also an area for concern, as evidence shows that both qualified nurses and trainee students are seriously lacking in basic numeracy skills.

This key book provides a guide to calculation skills and includes the core charts, prescription models, labels and diagrams (such as syringes) needed by student and practising nurses or midwifes.

Importantly this text will provide context through the use of senarios and examples that refer to all branches of nursing and midwifery.

*Contents: Basic mathematical skills – Fluid balance charts – Medications safety – Oral medications – Injections and IV fluids – More complex calculations for critical care areas.*

December 2008   152pp
978-0-335-23359-5 (Paperback)

# Clinical Skills

The Essence of Caring

**Helen Iggulden, Caroline Macdonald, Karen Staniland**

*Clinical Skills: The Essence of Caring* is an innovative new textbook and integrated Media Tool package which makes teaching and learning nursing interactive! Based on the Essence of Care, this book covers the core clinical skills curriculum and takes a holistic approach to the importance of delivering excellent nursing care.

Comprehensive coverage – an accessible account of all fundamental skills is provided, including Record Keeping, Communication and Pressure Ulcers.
Pedagogy – a multitude of activity and case study boxes, a glossary, self-test questions and 25 patient scenarios really bring the topics to life.
Inside every book is a free Media Tool DVD offering a wealth of fully integrated interactive material that is versatile enough to use in solo study, group assignments or classroom sessions. The DVD includes:

Case studies: This section contains a video case study for each nursing branch (Adult, Child, Mental Health and Learning Disability) which follows a patient journey to highlight the importance of empathic caring.

Skill Sets: This section includes video demonstrations and self-test questions for the clinical skills covered in first and second year nursing programmes, including: Infection Control, Wound Care, and Administration of Medicines.
Chapter Resources: This section contains extra supporting chapter material and includes questions, links, key learning resources and examples of both good and bad practice.

This comprehensive package offers a unique way of relating theory to practice, making it an essential learning resource for all CFP and nursing students.

*Contents – Clinical skills: the essence of caring – Communication – Record keeping – The care environment – Privacy and Dignity – Safety of patients with mental health needs – Self care – Personal and oral hygiene Food and nutrition – Continence, bladder and bowel care – Pressure ulcers*

2009   236pp
978-0-335- 23558 (Paperback)   978-0-335- 2356–5 (Hardback)